Pig Ailments

RECOGNITION AND TREATMENT

Mark White BVSc DPM MRCVS

Foreword by Dr Stanley Done

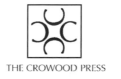

THE CROWOOD PRESS

First published in 2005 by
The Crowood Press Ltd
Ramsbury, Marlborough
Wiltshire SN8 2HR

www.crowood.com

British Library Cataloguing-in-Publication Data
A catalogue record for this book is available from the British Library.

ISBN 1 86126 787 8

Disclaimer
The author and the publisher do not accept responsibility in any manner
whatsoever for any error or omission, nor any loss, damage, injury or
liability of any kind incurred as a result of the use of any of the information
contained in this book, or reliance upon it.

Line drawings by Annette Findlay.

Acknowledgements
My thanks go to all those colleagues who over the years have provided
advice and guidance to steer me through the muddy waters of clinical
practice. In particular, special thanks go to Professor Dick Penny, Dr Tom
Alexander, Dr Bill Smith, John Oldham, Dr Stan Done, John Mackinnon,
John Wilkinson, Jill Thomson, David Chennells and the late Richard Potter.
I wish to apologize to them and others for flagrantly reproducing some of
their comments and ideas as my own. The exchange of slides over the years
has led to faded memories of ownership and I hope the original lenders
forgive me for using them.
    Finally, I would also like to thank the numerous pig farmers who have
provided me with the perfect learning environment and, without whom, this
book would not have been possible.

Typefaces used: Goudy (*text*), Cheltenham (*headings*).

Typeset and designed by D & N Publishing
Hungerford, Berkshire.

Printed and bound in Great Britain by CPI Bath.

Contents

Foreword

Mark White is more than capable of writing a preface to this very useful volume. Instead, he did me the honour of inviting me to write a foreword. It is with real pleasure that I agreed to this novel task.

Mark is eminently placed to write this book. As a pig practitioner, he was mentored by such notables as Ted Nelson and John Oldham, quite a tough apprenticeship in itself. Furthermore, he has been a member of the Pig Veterinary Society for a large number of years, contributing papers and clinical club presentations, serving on the executive and acting as the society's president. As the chief pig specialist and practitioner of the Haven Group, Mark has been 'in pigs' for more years than he probably cares to remember, and as a result he has come across most of the diseases normally seen in the UK and a few others like foot and mouth disease and classical swine fever that we did not anticipate. He has also written the pig section for most editions of the *UK Vet* periodical, has been a significant contributor to *In Practice*, sister journal of the *Veterinary Record*, and has done his share of 'scrutineering' articles for publication. Not least, of course, Mark's pig expertise has been recognized over the years by his association with breeding companies in his role as a company vet. A close interest in legal and medicinal matters has further honed his expertise.

One of the greatest skills required of a practitioner who is always short of time and beset by customers worried about costs is the ability to crystallize one's thoughts and get to the heart of the matter quickly. This great asset is possessed by Mark in abundance, as evident in this text, which is erudite, succinct and crystal-clear. It is therefore with great pleasure that Mark's friends and colleagues will receive this book, as they know it comes from a wealth of experience and with a considerable amount of expertise in all aspects of modern pig health and welfare. It can therefore be recommended unreservedly to all those in the industry who need a text that is both practical and concise. In addition, it concentrates on those items that are the key features of modern practitioner-oriented pig practice. The minutiae of nomenclature and laboratory-based diagnoses are not included (nor do they need to be), but the essence of clinical practice is explained succinctly. This highly readable book is a worthy successor to other books produced in the UK by a succession of eminent practitioners and will be invaluable in stimulating the next generation to come forward.

Dr Stanley Done,
BVetMed, BA, PhD,
DiplECVP, FRCVS

Introduction

The purpose of this book is to provide an easily accessible reference of the major diseases and abnormalities that occur in pigs. Although the descriptions are based upon experiences in the UK and Europe, they apply throughout the world and provide information that is relevant to large commercial pig herds, small hobby/backyard pig farming and pet-pig keepers. The target audience for the book is veterinary surgeons, veterinary students, experienced pig stockmen and pig owners.

Pig Ailments has been put together on the basis of twenty-five years of clinical experience working with pigs and, it is hoped, is presented in a practical and user-friendly format, with illustrations and photographs to aid explanation and recognition. It is not intended as a definitive scientific text – more technical information is available to those who require it from the sources listed in the Bibliography (*see* page 156). While every effort has been made to avoid too much technical terminology, a glossary is included on page 157.

The book is divided into two main parts. The first covers diseases of breeding animals – both the female and the male – and concentrates on the clinical problems that limit the successful breeding of the sow. While this section concerns both infectious diseases and managemental failures that lead to a shortfall in the productivity of the breeding herd, it is not written as a handbook of pig management. That said, managemental aspects are highlighted where they impact on the incidence and severity of disease.

The second section is devoted to ailments that are categorized by the effect they have on different body systems. It is hoped that this will allow easy referencing. For example, a problem that displays diarrhoea as its principal clinical sign is likely to be found within the section on enteric disease. Conversely, where coughing predominates, detail is likely to be found under respiratory tract diseases.

It is worth remembering here that the veterinary clinician is indebted to research scientists for providing the basis for understanding of how each disease works; only with that knowledge can he or she provide advice on treatments and control programmes.

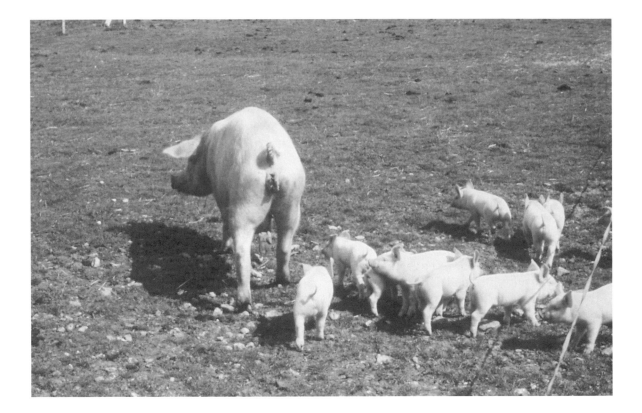

PART 1: Diseases of Breeding Animals

CHAPTER ONE

Diseases of Reproduction

In this first chapter, we will look at the foundations of pig production – reproduction and breeding. While it is often easy to blame disease when breeding problems arise, in very many cases the cause is managemental failure – in the broadest sense – rather than specific infection. There is therefore a need to apprcciate the link between fertility, reproduction and herd productivity. It is not the intention to cover the latter in any great detail – many other texts are available. Here, we will look at the overall breeding approach from a physiological point of view and illustrate how this is affected by management, housing, nutrition and disease.

PRODUCTION TARGETS AND BASIC PHYSIOLOGY

The ancient wild ancestors of modern farmed pigs were seasonal breeders, having a peak fertile period coinciding with short day length such that they would farrow in the spring some 115 days later. The modern pig breeds all year and, when not pregnant, has an oestrous cycle of twenty-one days (the normal range is eighteen to twenty-four days). There is, however, some residual seasonality in pig breeding, in that fertility tends to be lower in summer and autumn, and conversely litter size is at its maximum early in the year (in the northern hemisphere).

On a herd basis, reasonable targets for breeding success are a farrowing rate of 85 per cent – in other words, out of every 100 sows, 85 will farrow to that service. As a general rule, gilts and older sows will have lower success rates (75–80 per cent), indicating that the overall herd fertility will be affected by herd age structure. The farrowing rate is a measure of fertility. It is often confused with the farrowing index (the number of litters produced per sow per year), which is a measure of productivity. A reasonable target farrowing index for a commercial herd would be 2.35.

The breeding life of a sow is highly variable. Wild sows and pet/backyard sows that are not particularly productive can live and breed for at least ten years. However, farmed pigs tend to tail off in terms of fertility and productivity after six or seven litters, giving them a maximum age of three to four years. Many will be culled earlier than this as a result of disease,

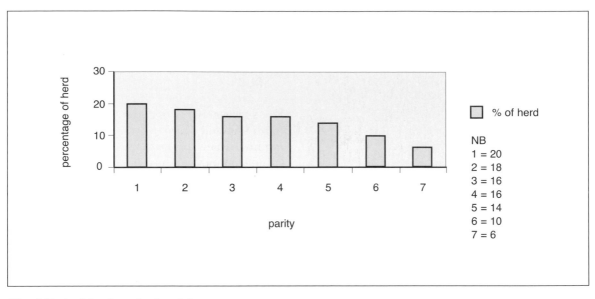

Fig. 1 Typical herd parity breakdown.

injury, non-breeding or low productivity. Thus, in a modern commercial herd, the average parity of the herd will be around three litters, reached by the age of two years.

Gilts are usually bred no earlier than seven months of age, although Chinese breed-types and their crosses can be bred successfully from five months. Puberty typically occurs from five to six months (in Chinese breed-types from four months plus), and optimum lifetime production can be achieved by serving gilts on their third cycle or beyond above the age of 210 days. There is a fall-off in fertility in gilts bred after the age of 260 days (in modern white breeds with or without Duroc blood).

Oestrus

For approximately thirty-six to forty-eight hours in each three-week cycle, the gilt or sow will be on heat and receptive to the boar; towards the end of this period ovulation will occur. Successful breeding depends on the correct detection of heat, or oestrus.

Signs of Oestrus

The signs of a pig on heat are easier to detect in the gilt than the sow, but care is needed to differentiate the period before standing oestrus (pro-oestrus) and the true heat. During pro-oestrus, appetite will drop, the vulva will become reddened and swollen, a small amount of mucus may be discharged and the gilt or sow will attempt to mount others (which will object). Pro-oestrus can last up to twenty-four hours, by which time the vulval swelling will start to subside, the animal will stand to be ridden with ears pricked – especially if back pressure is exerted – and a characteristic squeal may be emitted.

If a boar is available in fenceline contact, the oestrus animal will tend to stand close by for periods of time. Rather than be 'standing' continually over a period of thirty-six hours, as is the case with pro-oestrus animals, the oestrus gilt or sow will have many twenty- to thirty-minute episodes separated by one to three hours – in which she will stand to be mated or ridden. Oestrus can, therefore, be easy to miss if stockmen are not astute or experienced.

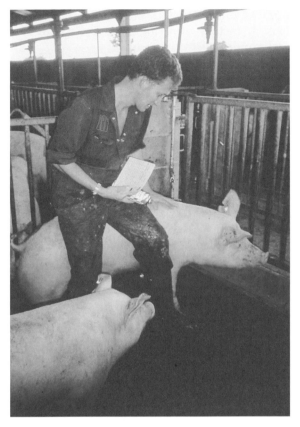

Fig. 2 Applying pressure to the back of a sow that is on heat will induce a standing response.

Oestrus in Gilts

In modern commercial breed types, puberty will occur from five months onwards, depending on stimulus. The primary stimulation arises from a boar and, in particular, from the pheromone androstenone he produces from his salivary glands. Intermittent boar contact is preferable, as continual contact tends to lead to habituation and a failure in the gilt to cycle. Other factors that will influence oestrus onset include the following:

1. Temperature and its effects on energy balance.
2. Nutrition.
3. Lighting levels – fourteen to sixteen hours of light within a 24-hour period are necessary, with sufficient intensity such that you can read close print.
4. Air quality – high ammonia levels will mask the pheromones, thereby reducing the 'boar effect'.

For successful cycling, the gilt will need to be in an anabolic state – in other words, on a rising nutritional plane while still growing. Anything that pushes the gilt into a negative energy balance (when she is burning up energy) will impede egg growth, oestrus onset and ovulation. Thus, while there are no disease conditions that specifically impede oestrus onset, any systemic illness that requires the mounting of an energy-expensive immune response will have this effect. Damage to the nasal chambers (for example, by atrophic rhinitis in the young gilt – *see* page 72) will reduce the likelihood of oestrus occurring, owing to reduced olfactory reception to boar pheromones.

Oestrus in Sows

During lactation, the sow produces a hormone called prolactin. Among other effects, this blocks the oestrous cycle and thus, in general (unlike in cattle and horses), sows will not show oestrus while lactating. The aim is to ensure that sows come on heat within seven days of weaning, although this will be influenced by a number of factors:

1. Weaning age. Sows weaned early (less than twenty-one days after farrowing) will tend to take longer to come on heat as the prolactin levels are at a peak during the third week of lactation. Sows with extended lactation lengths – either as a result of policy or through their use as foster mothers – may actually break through the prolactin block and cycle while lactating, especially if lactation exceeds thirty-five days. This may not be detected and will then push post-weaning oestrus to twenty-one days after lactational oestrus. Cycling in sows during lactation tends to be more of an issue in outdoor production where litter desertion can

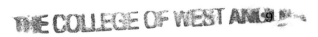

be common, effectively producing early weaning.

2. Energy balance. During lactation, the sow is likely to be in a catabolic state (a negative energy balance) due to the high demands of milk production. This is especially the case in younger sows, which are still growing. Following weaning, there will be an energy surge as milk production ceases, in turn leading to a rise in blood glucose levels. This induces a spike of insulin production, which sets off a cascade of hormones that induce the onset of oestrus in the absence of the prolactin block. Excessive weight loss during lactation and a failure to feed well after weaning, either by design or as a result of bullying in weaning yards, will therefore impede oestrus onset. Likewise, any excessive demands on energy after weaning – such as excessive cold and draughts, disease challenge, discomfort and stress – will also impede oestrus onset.

3. Boar contact. As with gilts, pheromones from the boar act to stimulate the sow's neuro-endocrine system and induce oestrus. Intermittent contact (thirty minutes in every twenty-four hours from the day of weaning) with a mature (at least fourteen months old) boar will be beneficial, or artificial pheromones (available in aerosol cans) can be administered if this is not possible.

4. Light levels. As with gilts, adequate lighting is essential for oestrus stimulation, particularly to override the seasonal effects of decreasing day length in late summer and autumn.

On a herd basis, the aim should be for an average weaning to first service interval of five days. However, sows should not be served between seven and ten days post-weaning as this period has been shown to be sub-fertile.

Litter Size

A newborn litter will contain, variably, live piglets, stillborn piglets (dealt with in more detail in Chapter 3) and mummified piglets. The aim of any pig farmer is to maximize the number of live piglets born, so here we will look at factors affecting total litter size and embryonic or foetal death.

Ovulation Rates

In the young gilt following puberty, the number of eggs released will increase in successive cycles (*see* Fig. 3). This is another good reason for not serving gilts until at least their third heat period. The various factors discussed above that influence oestrus onset in gilts and sows will also have an effect on ovulation rates. Thus, a strong positive energy balance as a result of a rising plane of nutrition is beneficial – this is often referred to as 'flushing'. Conversely, early weaning in sows will reduce ovulation rates. Genetic selection also plays a large part in determining ovulation rates, and over a number of years has produced hyperprolific lines. Herd age structure will, again, influence litter size as peak size occurs in sows that are between third and sixth parity.

Heat	Number of eggs released	Litter size
First heat	10–12	8
Second heat	12–15	9.5
Third heat	15–18	10.2

Fig. 3

Fertilization

Fertilization is the process by which the sperm penetrates the egg and the genetic material derived from dam and sire merges. Successful fertilization not only requires viable semen but correct timing of insemination, or service. Once eggs are released by the sow, they will last only six to eight hours before they begin to degenerate. Spermatozoa have to go through a maturation process, which occurs at the utero-tubular junction, before they are capable of penetrating the egg, a process that takes two hours. Therefore, the aim is to serve two hours prior to ovulation. The problem lies in establishing when ovulation occurs! Typically, it is said to occur twelve hours before the end of standing oestrus. In practice, however, the variability in oestrus length means that it is usual to serve two or three times at intervals of twelve to twenty-four hours throughout oestrus. The key to achieving maximum fertilization is to avoid late serving.

Conception
Following fertilization of the eggs, cell division takes place while the egg floats freely in the fallopian tube or uterine horn. From approximately ten days post-fertilization, the fertilized egg elongates and attaches to the wall of the uterus (this is often referred to – incorrectly – as implantation). Once attached, the embryos release a chemical signal to the sow to indicate their presence and this prevents the sow coming back on heat at three weeks. This is the process of conception. It is vital that sufficient chemical signal is sent by the embryos; as a general rule, at least four developing embryos are needed for this. If fewer embryos attach to the uterine wall, the signal will fail and the sow will return to heat at three weeks.

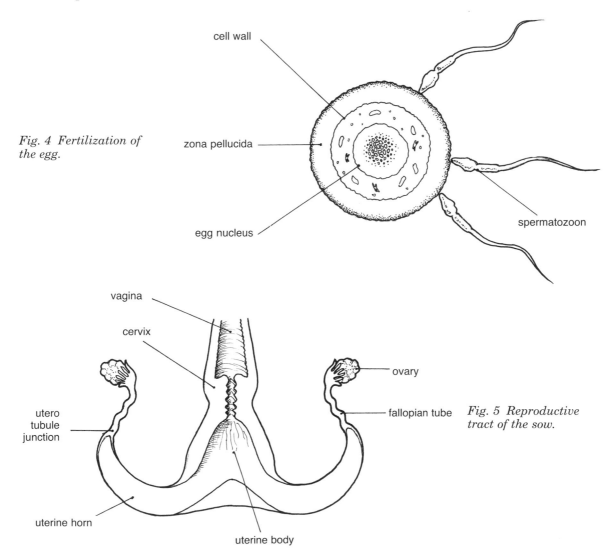

Fig. 4 Fertilization of the egg.

cell wall

zona pellucida

egg nucleus

spermatozoon

vagina

cervix

ovary

utero tubule junction

fallopian tube

uterine horn

uterine body

Fig. 5 Reproductive tract of the sow.

11

Embryonic Development

Differentiation of the embryo continues up until thirty to thirty-five days post-service, by which time the main body structures have formed (heart, lungs, intestine, liver, brain and so on), along with the placenta. However, between attachment (completed by fourteen to eighteen days post-service) and thirty-five days, it is possible for embryos to die for a wide range of reasons, so that litter size will decrease in some cases to fewer than four. Embryos that die before thirty-five days are reabsorbed, leaving no evidence of their existence. Despite this, pregnancy will still be maintained, even if there is only one developing embryo – it is only the death of all embryos that will lead to a return to service by the sow. Death of embryos may occur as a result of disease (for example, parvovirus – *see* page 13), genetic abnormality, asynchrony of fertilization (the production of embryos of varying ages that are not compatible) or stress and disruption to the sow.

Foetal Development

The period between 35 and 115 days gestation is marked by progressive growth of the foetus. The placenta – separate for each piglet – will grow until approximately sixty days gestation, while the skin and bone of the foetuses are laid down from thirty-five days onwards.

Death can occur to individual piglets at any stage, but because of the presence of the skeleton after thirty-five days, it is not possible for the foetus to be completely reabsorbed from this time on. In such cases only the fluid component will be reabsorbed, leaving a dried, mummified carcass (*see* Fig. 7). Death may be the result of infection (for example, parvovirus), placental insufficiency, insufficient uterine space (especially in large litters) or genetic abnormality. If the whole litter dies and becomes mummified, then the farrowing process will be stalled (*see* Chapter 2). However, in most cases death and mummification affect only a proportion of the developing litter, which are born along with live piglets. It is possible to estimate the stage of death of a mummified pig (days since service) by measuring the distance between the crown of the skull and the base of the tail (in centimetres) and then applying this to the following formula:

d = 3L + 20

where d is the days of gestation (age of the foetus) and L (cm) is the crown–rump length.

Pregnancy Failure

Pregnancy can fail at any time and usually results in a return to service. The time interval between service and return will be influenced by the stage at which loss of the litter occurs, and can be broken down into five categories:

1. Regular three-week returns. These will be seen if fertilization fails to occur, if fertilized eggs die within ten days and if conception fails totally (in other words, fewer than four embryos attach to the wall of the uterus).
2. Delayed (irregular) returns. If conception occurs, the signal is sent to the sow by the attached embryos. However, if they subsequently die, the sow will come back on heat at an abnormal time, often between twenty-eight and thirty-five days.
3. Regular six-week returns. Returns picked up at six weeks post-service are most likely to be three-week returns that were not spotted and, thus, have gone round another cycle.
4. Abortions. Complete loss of the litter beyond thirty-five days results either in whole litter mummification (and no returns to oestrus) or abortion. In the pig, abortion tends to occur most commonly in the third trimester (beyond seventy-five days gestation), although occasionally early embryonic loss may manifest as shedding of embryonic remnants (in other words, abortion) rather than reabsorption. Following abortion, a sow is likely to show oestrus within seven days. In a farm situation, abortion rates should not exceed 2 per cent per annum. As a rule of thumb, a sow or gilt that is seen

in oestrus beyond fifty days post-service can be regarded either as a return that was not seen earlier or as a result of abortion.

6. Anoestrus. In some cases, following loss of a litter at any stage, the sow's reproductive control mechanism will 'shut down' and she will not come on heat. This can also happen in maiden gilts (which may be permanently hormonally abnormal) and in weaned sows. Treatment with hormonal cocktails may assist. However, where a whole litter has died and become mummified, farrowing will not occur and the sow will not come on heat; in such cases prostaglandin treatment is needed to remove the litter.

SPECIFIC REPRODUCTION DISEASES

The vast majority of diseases relevant to this section are specific to the pregnant sow and the effects her infection will have on the unborn litter. Where systemic disease in the sow occurs (such as with erysipelas – *see* page 16), interference with oestrus onset and fertilization can occur, but this is an indirect effect that is caused primarily by the negative energy balance of the sow.

Porcine Parvovirus (PPV)

Apart from a single very unusual report of skin disease in weaners, PPV is solely associated with reproductive failure or with its effect on an unborn litter. Infection of the non-pregnant animal has no clinical effect and immunity is acquired that will be life-long and will protect all future litters. The effects that PPV infection will have on a pregnant sow depend on the stage of pregnancy and are summarized in Figure 6 below. From this it can be seen that the effects of PPV infection can be **s**tillbirth, **m**ummification, **e**mbryonic **d**eath and **i**nfertility, giving the old acronym SMEDI. It should be noted that abortion is a very rare manifestation of PPV infection.

On a herd basis, in a naive herd, an outbreak of PPV disease will last two to three months and will be manifest by varying signs over that time in the following sequence:

1. Increased regular returns to oestrus lasting two to three weeks.
2. Increased irregular returns to oestrus lasting two to three weeks simultaneously with above.
3. Stillborn pigs starting simultaneously with above for one to two months.

Stage of reproductive cycle	Effect of PPV infection	Result
Non-pregnant	No effect	Immunity
At service and within 10 days of service	Death of fertilized eggs/differentiating embryos	Return to service at three weeks
10–25 days post-service	Embryonic death	Delayed return to service or small litter
25–75 days post-service	Foetal death, often progressive through the litter	Variable-sized mummified pigs affecting whole or part of the litter, and/or stillborn pigs
75 days plus	Minimum effect on foetuses as immune response can be raised	Possibly small pigs born that have been checked during growth, and stillborn pigs

Fig. 6 Effect of PPV infection on pregnant sows.

4. Increase in mummified pigs from six to twelve weeks after (1) above, and failures to farrow.
5. Drop in total litter size for two to three weeks from eighty days after start of the outbreak.

It is, thus, a sequential disease, the classic sign of which is large numbers of mummified pigs within litters, of variable size, starting around one month after an increase in returns to service. The diagnosis of PPV disease is based on the clinical picture supported by serological testing using an haemagglutination inhibition test or ELISA test, and by virus detection in the livers of mummified or stillborn pigs.

Prevention and Control
Highly effective vaccines against PPV are available worldwide and are given to gilts prior to breeding. The actual programme (number of doses and timing) varies between products, but it should be noted that maternally derived antibodies (those passed to a piglet in colostrum) can survive for up to six months and that these can block vaccine efficacy. Vaccination should, therefore, not be given too early in life. Vaccine protocols often advocate repeated dosing throughout life (either after every litter or every other litter), but in practice this is rarely necessary since field virus acts to boost immunity imparted from gilt vaccination. This can be verified by serological monitoring of a herd on a biannual basis.

An alternative prevention method where vaccines are not available is the unreliable technique of feedback, whereby weaner faeces derived from pigs eight to ten weeks of age are offered to gilts for the period four to two weeks before intended service. This method is based

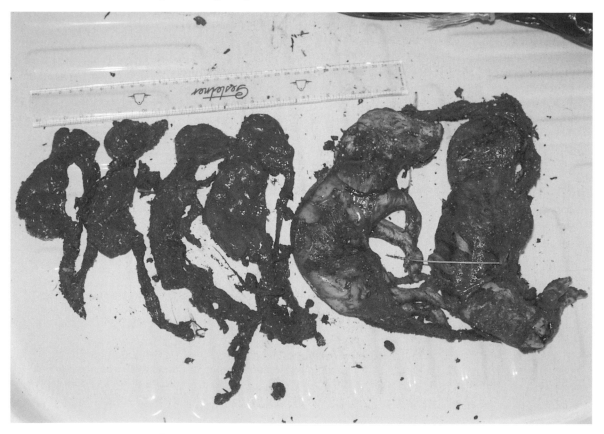

Fig. 7 Progressive mummification resulting from porcine parvovirus (PPV) infection.

on the presumption that some excretion of virus occurs from this age group.

RELATED DISEASES

Before the identification of the porcine parvovirus, the syndrome it causes was described as SMEDI. It is now known that most outbreaks of this disease are due to PPV infection, although there are several enteroviruses that can, on rare occasions, produce the identical syndrome and so should always be considered, especially in herds vaccinated for PPV. There are no vaccines available for this group of viruses and control rests in the technique of feeding back infected material to maiden gilts during an outbreak in countries where this is permissible (the practice is not allowed in the UK).

Porcine Reproductive and Respiratory Syndrome (PRRS)

Here, PRRS is discussed solely with reference to its effects on reproduction; other manifestations of this viral infection are discussed in Chapters 6, 7 and 10.

In primary PRRS breakdowns affecting naive herds, it is common to see a rise in returns to service, although it is unclear whether this is a direct effect on the unborn litter or the result of systemic illness in the sow affecting ovulation, fertilization or conception/embryonic attachment. The principal specific reproductive effects tend to occur in the third trimester, and cause abortion, premature farrowing, late mummification, stillbirths and birth of extremely weak piglets. This may or may not be accompanied by illness in the sow.

The European strains of PRRS virus tend to produce a relatively mild outbreak, although

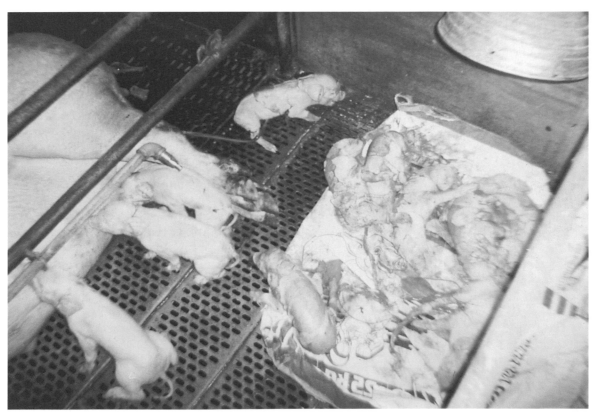

Fig. 8 Weak and stillborn pigs following in utero *porcine reproductive and respiratory syndrome (PRRS) infection.*

piglet mortality as a result of weakness at birth and subsequent disease can reach 50 per cent over a period of six to eight weeks. Abortion rates rarely exceed 5 per cent but can grumble on within a herd for years. Unlike PPV disease, which tends to be epizootic and explosive but disappears after three months, PRRS will often cause permanent or recurrent disease in a herd. Occasional strains of PRRS identified in North America can be far more dramatic. These produce abortion storms affecting 50 per cent of pregnant sows and also result in very high sow mortality rates. These specific strains have not been seen in Europe, although other US strains are known.

Prevention and Control
Historically, gilts entering a farm as replacements have been at the root of PRRS problems. In some cases, they may enter in a naive state, pick up infection and then act as generators, causing the virus to reinfect the sow herd. Where gilts enter as 'positive' animals, they may be excretors of virus – possibly of a different strain to that on the farm – again, causing destabilization. It is therefore essential that incoming gilts are isolated and allowed to settle before they mix with indigenous sows and boars, thereby ensuring they are exposed to the virus in isolation. This can be achieved erratically by exposure to weaner faeces or to live twelve-week-old weaners for at least a month, but vaccines – both live and dead – are available variably in Europe and North America. Difficulties have, however, been encountered with live North American strain vaccines, which are capable of both producing disease in vaccinated animals and replicating and spreading out. This has not been the case with live European strains. However, in Europe the choice of vaccination will depend on strain identification (North American strains are present here) and the balance between the increased risk of using a live vaccine against their claim of better efficacy over killed vaccines.

It is worth noting that boars infected with PRRS virus as a primary infection can excrete the virus in semen for many weeks. They can thus be a source of spread, either on farm or from artificial insemination (AI) studs to other customer farms.

Aujeszky's Disease (AD), or Pseudorabies
Aujeszky's disease is another viral (herpes virus) disease of pigs and other species, which has a wide range of effects that include reproductive failure in breeding stock as well as respiratory and nervous disease in young and growing pigs. The effect is both systemic, producing inappetance, lethargy and respiratory disease in the sow, as well as specific, causing abortion, mummification and stillborn pigs (these may be putrefying and macerated). In a naive population, abortions can occur in up to 50 per cent of affected sows. The disease does affect other animal species (although man is resistant), and a frequent occurrence on actively affected farms is the death of farm dogs and cats.

Prevention and Control
AD has been eradicated from some European countries and regions (for example, Denmark and Great Britain), while in many other western European countries control programmes are in place with a view to eliminating the virus. These programmes use a combination of vaccination and test and removal procedures. Outside of Europe, the disease is widespread in North and South America and Asia. Both live and inactivated vaccines are available, although gene-detected vaccines are particularly popular as they enable differentiation between a vaccinated animal and one that has been exposed to field virus. A feature of natural infection with AD virus – as with all herpes viruses – is long-term carriage and repeated or perpetual excretion, a situation that does not occur in vaccinated animals.

Erysipelas
The major reproductive feature of erysipelas is abortion, usually in later pregnancy, and it is generally associated with illness in the sow,

including high rectal temperatures (in excess of 41°C/106°F). It is possible on the farm to see only this manifestation of the disease – in other words, infection need not necessarily be the result of a major outbreak of erysipelas in growing pigs. The causative bacteria *Erysipelothrix rhusiopathiae* (which has also been called *Erysipelas insidiosa*) is ubiquitous and, in particular, is commonly carried and excreted by wild birds and rodents. The organism can usually easily be grown from aborted foetuses and is probably one of the most common causes of definitively diagnosed abortion in the sow.

Prevention and Control
Serotypes 1 and 2 are the most commonly found disease-causing strains of the bacteria and are covered by vaccines, all of which contain serotype 2 and some of which contain serotype 1 as well. Although immunity from vaccination is not long-lasting, a thorough vaccination programme involving two-dose primary courses and booster doses within six months throughout life is usually effective at preventing clinical disease in sows.

It is worth pointing out here one of the problems arising from the use of the feedback method (*see* page 60) to treat infections such as rotavirus. In this method the sow is exposed to natural infection – usually infected faeces – to stimulate immunity. It is, however, possible to create and perpetuate an outbreak of erysipelas reproductive disease via farrowing-house faeces through its contact with late pregnant sows. Where the feedback technique is used, it is therefore essential that it ceases immediately should any signs of erysipelas appear in sows.

Endometritis/Vaginitis
The vagina of the sow is bacteriologically contaminated, mostly with environmental- and faecal-based organisms. In addition, such bacteria as *Streptococcus suis* and *Arcanobacterium pyogenes* (formerly *Actinomyces pyogenes*) are common colonizers of the vagina. The cervix acts as a doorway to the uterus, keeping these

bacteria out. The prepuce and preputial diverticulum of the boar are also heavily contaminated with similar microflora. Whenever the cervix is open, it is therefore possible for bacteria to ascend into the uterus, the most likely times being at farrowing (whence they should be flushed out) and at service or insemination.

The environment within the uterus during the early and middle stages of oestrus is extremely hostile to bacteria and any introduction at this time is unlikely to lead to colonization of the uterus. However, as oestrus subsides, the uterine environment becomes less hostile and any introduction is more likely to become established. The principal concerns here, therefore, are when serving occurs late in oestrus, and when infection is allowed to ascend in a heavily contaminated vagina before the cervix fully closes.

The effects of uterine contamination can be twofold:

1. It can set off an endometritis, which will preclude the successful attachment of embryos at ten to fourteen days post-service. This will lead to service either at three weeks or delayed to around four weeks, usually preceded in the two or three days beforehand by a purulent discharge. Severely contaminated sows may return to oestrus several times with a discharge.
2. Some organisms causing contamination (such as *Arcanobacterium pyogenes*) are ovicidal, and returns to oestrus after infection in these cases will occur at three weeks, without a discharge, as a result of a complete failure of fertilization.

It is also possible, particularly in older sows where vaginal contamination is excessive, for ascending bacteria to pass into the vagina as the cervix begins to relax and open in the week preceding farrowing. In some circumstances, this will kill the litter, which will be entirely stillborn and partially decomposing. Hygiene is critical to control this syndrome, particularly in confined sows where solid backboards allow faecal build-up. Equally, heavily contaminated

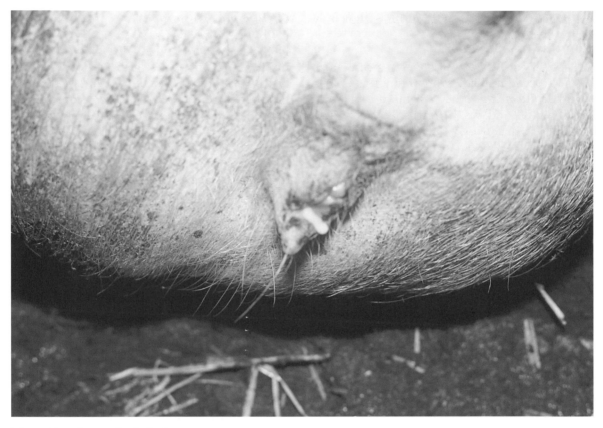

Fig. 9 Purulent vulval discharge.

weaning pens can contribute to vaginal colonization, while other factors linked to this syndrome include high manual intervention rates
at farrowing. It has also been speculated that a
high incidence of vulva damage due to biting
may be associated with increased levels of vaginal contamination and subsequent discharge-
associated infertility. Dirty insemination technique is also implicated.

Prevention and Control
Antimicrobial therapy is widely used to control such problems and can be administered
by a wide range of methods, including the following:

1. In-feed medication, although high inclusion
   levels are needed – for example, 1kg of
   chlorotetracycline per tonne of food.

2. Injection given at service.
3. Direct instillation of antibiotics into the
   anterior vagina after final mating.
4. Preputial washing/antibiotic instillation on
   a regular basis for boars.

The antibiotics most commonly used include
tetracyclines, tylosin and potentiated
sulphonamides. Culling of chronically affected
animals may be the only option in some cases.
As a general rule, artificial insemination is
associated with fewer discharge-related returns
to service than natural service, although it does
not eliminate the problems altogether.

Leptospirosis
Leptospira spp. are bacteria found widely in
pig and animal populations that are associated with reproductive failure in sows. There

are two major groups of *Leptospira* that may be implicated:

1. *Leptospira pomona*. This species can cause widespread and severe reproductive losses, particularly late abortion, mummification, stillbirths and weak piglets at birth. The sow will frequently be pyrexic following infection, evident by inappetance and lethargy. *L. pomona* is widespread in North America, Asia, Oceania and south and eastern Europe, but the classic pathogenic strains have never been found in the UK.

2. *Leptospira australis* group including *L. bratislava*. Statistical correlation between seropositive animals and infertility identified in the 1980s first raised the possibility of pathology associated with the *L. australis* group. The organism has been implicated in outbreaks of discharge-associated returns to service and can be found at the utero-tubular junction of affected animals. It has also been associated with abortion and has been identified by fluorescent antibody tests (FAT) in livers of aborted pigs.

Prevention and Control
Low-titre serological-positive sows can commonly be found in most herds, but this does not constitute a diagnosis of disease and it is likely that *Leptospira australis* is often over-diagnosed as a cause of infertility. In cases where a definitive diagnosis is achieved, gilts with unestablished herds seem to be most susceptible. In these instances, the use of antibiotics – either in feed (for example, tetracyclines) or by injection (for example, streptomycin) – are highly effective treatments.

Leptospira spp. can pass through semen, and so where a herd outbreak is confirmed the treatment of boars (with streptomycin) is indicated. Semen from commercial AI studs normally has antibiotics included to destroy any *Leptospira* contamination. Wildlife, including rats, mice and hedgehogs, can act as carriers and vectors of the *L. australis* group.

Chlamydophora
Chlamydophora spp. of bacterium (particularly *C. pecorum* and *C. trachomatis*) have been implicated in infertility outbreaks, particularly in Germany, producing a syndrome indistinguishable from endometritis/vaginitis. It is possible that cases of vaginal discharge and increase in returns to service that respond to tetracycline medication are involved with *Chlamydophora*. It should be noted that these organisms are zoonotic, as are those causing erysipelas and leptospiras, and so precautions should be taken. This is particularly important for women working on a pig farm, especially if they are of child-bearing age.

Prevention and Control
Control relies on the same approaches detailed above for endometritis/vaginitis.

Brucella suis
This is another serious bacterial disease of pigs that has reproductive implications. Early pregnancy infection leads to early abortion, reabsorption and delayed return to oestrus, while infection in late pregnancy tends to produce mummified, stillborn or weakened pigs, with copious bloody discharge associated with endometritis and placentitis. Infection can also cause testicular swelling (orchitis) in the boar and resultant sterility, and infected boars will pass the disease on to sows at service. (Bone and joint infections are other symptoms.)

A number of biotypes (strains) exist, some of which are geographically distinct – biotype 2, for example, is found only in western and central Europe, while biotype 3 is restricted to Asia and the Americas. In Europe, the European hare acts as an asymptomatic carrier and reservoir of biotype 2 and, as such, outdoor and feral pigs are at greatest risk.

Prevention and Control
Treatment of affected individuals is not very effective and slaughter policies are most widely employed. Vaccines have been produced and may be available in Asia. *Brucella suis* infection is notifiable within the European Union.

The related bacteria *B. abortus* (cattle) and *B. melitensis* (goats) are well recognized zoonoses, although *B. suis* appears to have a low affinity for man.

Other Exotic Reproductive Diseases

A wide range of infectious agents have been implicated in reproductive disease around the world, including toxoplasmosis, Japanese B encephalitis, encephalomyocarditis virus, classical and African swine fever, Nipah virus and paramyxovirus (blue eye). In general, other signs of these will be seen on farm in addition to infertility and abortion, but each must be included in any differential diagnosis of PRRS or Aujeszky's disease.

ADDITIONAL CAUSES OF REPRODUCTIVE PROBLEMS

Mycotoxins

A wide range of mycotoxins can affect feed and water, and they can have various effects on pigs of all ages. Of important note in the context of reproduction is zearalenone, an oestrogen mimic that can occur on spoilt maize in particular. In extreme cases, it can produce nymphomania, with sows appearing to be permanently on heat. At a lower level, high return rates to oestrus are seen and, in particular, the return can occur earlier than three weeks. The correct storage of feedstuffs and the destruction of any spoilt feed, especially that containing maize, is fundamental to the avoidance of such problems.

Nutrition

As discussed earlier in this chapter, major nutrient deficiency has a significant effect on reproduction and productivity. There are, however, numerous specific micronutrients that are essential to successful reproduction, including folic acid, biotin and vitamin A, a shortage of which will lead to reproduction problems. Furthermore, certain foodstuffs are known to contain chemicals classified as anti-nutrients – but which could be regarded as poisons – that have specific deleterious effects on reproduction. Eruscic acid and glucosinolates found in many oil-seed products such as rape meal and mustard-seed meal are specific examples of these, and levels of such meals in breeding diets must therefore be limited to avoid problems. (Note, however, that modern varieties of oil-seed rape – the so-called 'double zero' varieties – are bred specifically to reduce levels of these chemicals.)

To conclude, infectious disease is often blamed for reproductive and productivity problems on the farm. In reality, however, management, stockmanship and environment are frequently more significant, and the full investigation of production by way of detailed breeding records is therefore necessary to unravel most problems. Diagnostic testing should form only part of an investigation and serology should be viewed with extreme caution as a diagnostic tool for agents known to be enzootic within pig populations.

CHAPTER TWO

Parturition

Having discussed the establishment of pregnancy and the major diseases of reproduction, we now turn our attention to the farrowing process. In this chapter, the normal patterns will be discussed along with the major causes of problems. Brief description is provided of the technique required where interference is indicated.

INITIATION

Gestation in the sow lasts 115 ±3 days and, in common with all mammalian species, parturition (farrowing) is triggered not by the sow herself but by the litter. As the developing foetuses grow and reach a point where the space becomes limited in the uterus, the shortage of both oxygen and food (sugar) creates a 'stress' in them. They release corticosteroid hormones, which act as a trigger mechanism for a hormonal cascade that leads to the release, by the sow, of prostaglandins. The prostaglandins in turn destroy the structures on the ovaries (corpora lutea) that normally produce the hormone progesterone, which maintains pregnancy.

As a general rule, the larger the litter the earlier this stress will occur, and so sows carrying large litters tend to farrow earlier. Conversely, if only one live pig is present, farrowing may be delayed as the trigger mechanism is minimized. Moreover, if the whole litter has died and been mummified, there will be no signal and hence no farrowing (if the whole litter dies late and putrefies, however, the toxins released will themselves act as a trigger).

NORMAL FARROWING

The time from start of farrowing to completion is highly variable, with a range of one to eight hours (the former only if one or two pigs are present), although a 'normal' picture is of three to four hours for a litter of ten to twelve pigs. Following production of the litter, the placenta will usually be shed as a single mass within the hour. However, in some cases placenta may be shed part of the way through the farrowing process, an event that can normally be put down to the sow 'emptying one side' before starting on the other. (The placenta will often be stained with deposits of white urea, which is of no pathological consequence.)

The actual act of delivery of the pigs is controlled by the release of pulses of oxytocin

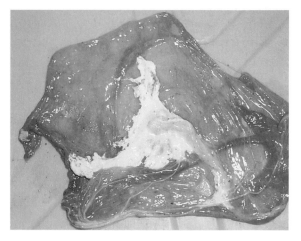

Fig. 10 Uric acid deposits on the placenta (normal).

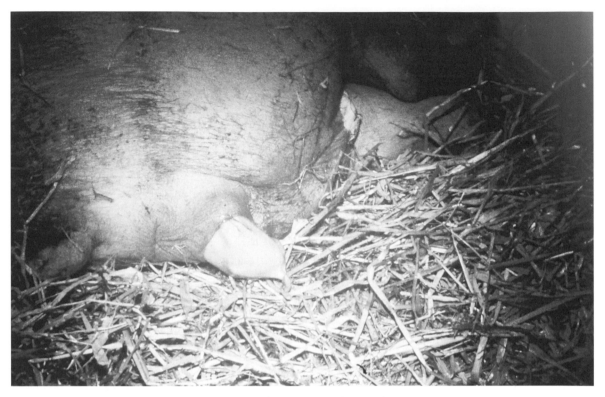

Fig. 11 Unassisted delivery of a piglet. The sow is in lateral recumbency.

Order of delivery	Time	Interval	Outcome
1	8.04am		Alive
2	8.18am	14 minutes	Alive
3 and 4	9.45am	87 minutes	Both alive
5	10.15am	30 minutes	Alive
6	10.32am	17 minutes	Alive
7	10.55am	23 minutes	Alive
8	12 noon	65 minutes	Stillborn
9	12.10pm	10 minutes	Alive
10 and 11	12.25pm	15 minutes	1 alive, 1 mummified
12	12.48pm	13 minutes	Alive
13	13.05pm	17 minutes	Stillborn and placenta
Total	**5 hours 1 minute**		**10 born alive;** **2 born dead;** **1 mummified**

Fig. 12 Typical sequence of piglet delivery in a fifth parity sow.

from the brain, which creates a wave of contraction in the uterine musculature (myometrium), effectively 'milking' the piglets out. Straining is not a prominent feature in the sow and delivery is usually preceded by fidgeting, frantic wagging of the tail and fluid discharge. Most sows will deliver pigs while lying on their sides. A failure of oxytocin release or a failure of the uterus to react to it has serious consequences for the birth of piglets.

While farrowing may last several hours, piglets do not tend to be produced at regular intervals. Figure 12 describes the delivery of one typical litter, which can be used as a model for many. The particular features to note are as follows:

1. Sows will often start to farrow, produce two or three piglets and then stop for anything up to 1½–2 hours without apparent ill-effects to subsequent piglets. 'Normal' farrowing intervals in the example used in Figure 12 were twenty to thirty minutes between piglets.
2. A delay in the second half of farrowing of more than thirty minutes appears to be associated with subsequent stillborn pigs. This pattern should be borne in mind when considering intervention. It is advisable for all farms to ascertain the 'normal' pattern of farrowings for their herd and, in particular, to note the variations between sows of different ages. As a general rule, gilts will farrow quicker (provided there are no obstructions) while older sows will tend to show the pattern described in Figure 12, with prolonged 'rest' periods.

CHEMICAL INTERFERENCE

Induction
It is possible to induce farrowing using prostaglandins given by injection, either for sows that are overdue (and hence the whole litter may be dead or mummified) or as a management tool to ensure sows farrow when attention is available. However, prostaglandin effects are not precisely predictable. Normally,

they will take between twenty-four and thirty-six hours to work, but a sow that has already started the chemical cascade may farrow before this time (in other words, the injected prostaglandin will have been redundant).

Injection is normally given into the muscle of the neck, although it can be more reliable if injected into the rump. Some producers inject half-doses into the inner wall of the vulva, although injection sterility is vital if this route is selected. To improve the predictability of farrowing following injection of prostaglandin, a follow-up injection of 10IU oxytocin can be given thirty hours after the prostaglandin to sows that have not started farrowing. The farrowing process will then commence within ninety minutes and will usually follow a stop-start pattern that then requires additional inference.

There are a number of rules that apply to the use of prostaglandins:

1. Never inject a sow of uncertain farrowing date and avoid use in herds where there is a habit of sows farrowing three weeks late (in other words, missed returns to service).
2. Induce sows to farrow no more than twenty-four hours before expected (in other words, inject at minus two days or minus one day).
3. Assess herd average gestation length before starting an induction programme.
4. Take note of individual sows with a history of delayed farrowing.
5. As a general rule, do not induce gilts that have highly variable gestation lengths.
6. Prostaglandins are dangerous to asthmatics and women of childbearing age – such people should not handle them.
7. Wear protective gloves when handling prostaglandins.

In theory, cortisone could be used to trigger farrowing by mimicking the piglet effect. However, the use of such chemicals is highly unpredictable and unreliable, and their use has largely been superseded by prostaglandin.

Delaying Parturition

Occasionally, there may be good reason to delay farrowing. This can be achieved using anti-prostaglandins such as aspirin (acetylsalicylic acid), or extraneous progesterone or progestogens. The licensing provision of such products – which will vary from country to country – should be noted in advance as this may affect the subsequent ability to slaughter for human consumption.

DYSTOCIA

Abnormal and interrupted farrowing is referred to as dystocia and results from a range of causes in the sow.

Maternal Dystocia

Uterine inertia is by far the most common cause of dystocia in the sow and is the result of a failure of the uterine muscle to contract and expel the piglets. It can arise in a number of circumstances:

1. As a temporary issue delaying farrowing, particularly in the later stages of the farrowing process, as shown in Figure 12.
2. In older sows where muscle tone is weakened or lost. The uterus can be thought of in the same light as a child's balloon – the more often it is blown up, the greater the degree of stretching, such that it never returns to its original form. The stretching of the muscle causes irreparable damage that reduces its ability to contract in future litters.
3. Calcium deficiency. Overt deficiency of calcium is rare in the modern commercial sow fed on well-formulated rations. Calcium is essential for muscle contraction and, when lacking, can cause inertia. An imbalance between calcium and phosphorous levels can also upset muscle contractility (*see also* 'Puffer Sows' on page 27).
4. Excessive body condition and lack of fitness. Overfat sows have much slower farrowings owing to poorer muscle contractility. It is also believed that inactivity – as occurs in confinement systems – has an effect on uterine tone at farrowing. Certainly, inertia appears far less common in free-range sows.
5. Adrenalin. Oxytocin is the effector of muscle contraction in the uterus. High levels of adrenalin are directly antagonistic to the effects of oxytocin and this is seen most commonly in 'hysterical' gilts crated for the first time. Rough handling that induces fear and excitement in sows can have similar effects.
6. Exhaustion/emaciation. Very thin sows lose the ability to contract muscle efficiently.
7. Overheating as a result of excessive environmental temperature will reduce uterine contractions.
8. Stresses resulting in high levels of circulating corticosteroids will reduce muscle tone and delay farrowing. Oversized sows squashed into farrowing crates are typically prone to this condition.

Prevention and Treatment

It is obviously vital to ensure that body condition is satisfactory at farrowing time in order to avoid excesses in either direction. Quiet handling and the crating of sows and, especially, gilts, well before farrowing is due (five days minimum) will reduce the risks of inertia. Attention to diet is likewise critical, and if inertia is a herd problem, biochemical analysis for blood calcium and phosphorus levels at the time of farrowing may indicate the cause. The injection of extraneous calcium can correct immediate problems in such cases.

The most useful corrective measure when farrowing has halted owing to inertia is the incremental use of oxytocin by injection. However, care is needed. If a large dose of oxytocin (10–20IU) is given in one go, a dramatic contraction will occur, expelling several piglets (provided there is no obstruction). However, the uterus will remain in spasm, such that unborn piglets become trapped above the contraction and will not be able to be delivered until the muscle has relaxed. This can take two to three hours. Moreover, at doses higher than this, the uterine contraction can be so violent that the uterus ruptures. When oxytocin is used to stimulate uterine contraction it is therefore essential to follow the guidelines below:

1. Use very small doses at a time (2–3IU) and repeat at intervals of twenty to thirty minutes as necessary.
2. Ensure there is no obstruction to delivery before administering oxytocin – either by manual examination (*see* 'Farrowing Intervention' below) or general observation of the sow. Never administer oxytocin to a sow or gilt that is visibly straining but failing to deliver.
4. Inject oxytocin into the muscle – the rump often gives better response than the neck.
5. Avoid the use of other uterine contractants such as ergometrine.

Foetal Dystocia

This is far less common than uterine inertia and results in an obstruction to the birth canal and consequent failure to deliver. Straining in the sow or gilt is the most prominent feature. Several situations where this is the case are seen:

1. Oversize piglet. Most commonly seen in gilts, either where litters are small (and hence piglets are large) or where the pelvis is abnormally and developmentally very narrow (this can run in families). The obstructing piglet will need to be removed manually or, if this is not possible, surgery is required.
2. Double presentation. Occasionally, two piglets may enter the uterine horn, cervix and vagina together – possibly when one piglet is released from either horn simultaneously. Manual removal is necessary in such cases.
3. Monsters. Various abnormalities of foetal development can occur, such as schistosoma reflexus and Siamese (conjoined) twins, and as with oversized piglets they can obstruct the birth canal. Manual removal or surgery is needed.

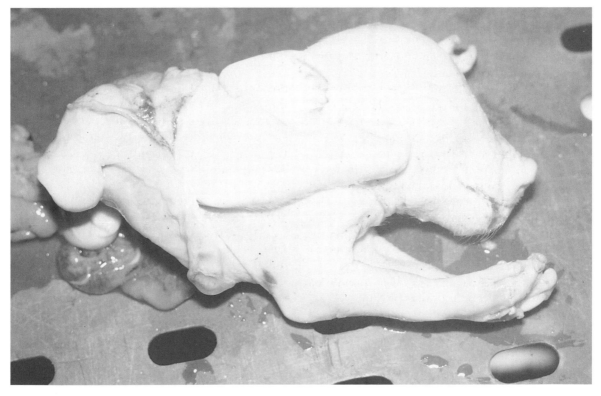

Fig. 13 Schistosoma reflexus.

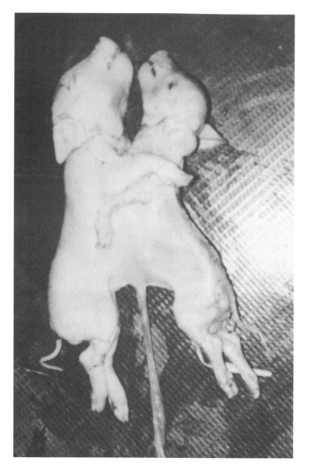

ABOVE: *Fig. 14 Conjoined (Siamese) pigs.*

Fig. 15 Piglet entrapment at the pelvic brim.

4. Pelvic brim obstruction. The gravid (pregnant) uterus hangs down into the abdomen from the pelvis, so the piglet has to pass over the pelvic brim during birth. It is possible, particularly in older sows, for the piglet's head to become trapped under the pelvic brim, blocking delivery. Often, such an obstruction can be released simply by getting the sow to her feet and walking her around. Otherwise, manual interference is needed.

OTHER FARROWING COMPLICATIONS

Prolapse

Vaginal prolapse can be quite common, particularly in tethered sows. In these instances the weight of the sow drops back to weaken the muscles of the perineum, thus prolapsing the vagina. This can obstruct farrowing.

Treatment

If the prolapse occurs well before farrowing is due, it can be replaced and sutures inserted across the vulva to keep it *in situ*. The sutures should be placed inside the vulva (in other words, through the mucosal lining) rather than

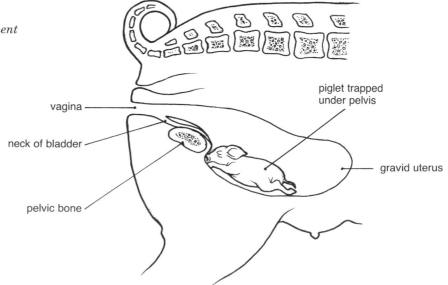

vagina

neck of bladder

pelvic bone

piglet trapped under pelvis

gravid uterus

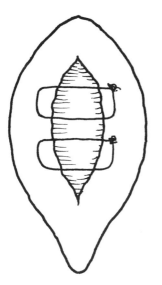

Fig. 16 Sutures laid across vulval lips,

through the outside skin to reduce subsequent straining. They must be removed prior to farrowing.

Where the prolapse is present at farrowing, it can be reduced by raising the back end of the sow on a board elevated on bricks (aim for 20–30cm/8–12in of elevation). This is clearly only possible in a farrowing crate.

Rarely, the bladder may displace backwards into the prolapse. In this position, the bladder cannot empty but will still be filled, and thus will get larger and larger. A failure to release the urine and replace the bladder will be fatal. Release can be achieved either by catheterization (difficult) or by draining through a large-bore needle, taking care to observe aseptic precautions (*see* Fig. 137 on page 150).

On some occasions, the cervix will prolapse out of the vagina prior to farrowing and appear as a large pink cauliflower. Such prolapses are difficult to replace and the sow may die as a result of internal rupture of the uterine artery.

Uterine Prolapse
Eversion of the entire uterus can occur at the end of farrowing and appears as two distinct horns outside the body. The uterus is very friable and prone to damage, and death due to shock can occur within two hours.

If the prolapse is spotted early and in an undamaged form, attempts can be made to replace it, although this is a difficult and frequently unsuccessful procedure. Techniques described include hoisting the sow by her back legs, filling the reinverting uterus with water or simple manipulation. Surgical amputation can be quick and effective, but severe blood loss can cause fatal shock (fluid or blood replacement is essential). In the commercial situation, rapid euthanasia is indicated. Such animals are not fit to be transported to a slaughterhouse.

Puffer Sows
This condition is occasionally seen in the immediate pre-farrowing period, when the sow will lie in sternal recumbancy in obvious distress and with a very high respiratory (and heart) rate and an elevated temperature. The condition can be fatal.

Treatment
While the clinical signs bear some similarities with eclampsia in the dog, there is no definitive evidence that this condition is an acute calcium deficiency. Equally, it is not necessarily part of the porcine stress syndrome (*see* page 141). The true cause remains unknown. However, if detected early, the following actions can be life-saving:

1. Hosing with cold water to reduce temperature.
2. Forced rebreathing by holding a paper bag over the head of the sow for three to four minutes (this may need repeating).
3. Use of tranquillizers.
4. Treatment with calcium borogluconate (CaBG) – 200ml of 40 per cent CaBG by intra-peritoneal injection.

Farrowing Intervention
Where an obstruction is suspected or oxytocin has failed to induce delivery of a piglet as a result of inertia, manual assistance must be given. The two golden rules that must always be followed are cleanliness and gentleness. The procedure follows the stages below:

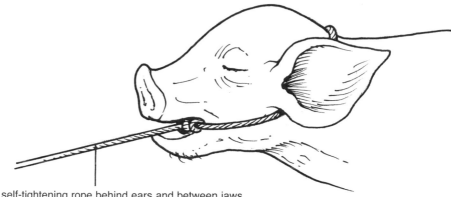

Fig. 17 Assisted delivery using rope.

self-tightening rope behind ears and between jaws

1. The sow should be adequately restrained, either lying on her side or standing (she is likely to move during interference).
2. The vulva and perineum should be thoroughly cleaned with warm water and dried with tissues.
3. Hands and arms must be thoroughly washed and arm-length gloves worn (these are as much to protect the operator from zoonotic infections as to protect the sow from contamination).
4. Liberal amounts of obstetrical lubricant should be applied to the hand, arm and vulval lips.
5. The hand should be formed into a cone and inserted into the vagina in a forwards and upwards direction.
6. The arm should be steadily and gently inserted until a piglet is found. In a big sow, a full arm length may be needed.
7. The piglet can be then extracted by placing fingers over its head (either side of the ears), by placing a finger in its mouth and grabbing the snout with the rest of the fingers, or by locking its legs between the fingers (especially if the piglet is in a backward presentation). If the piglet is tightly wedged, a sterile loop of rope can be fed behind the ears and between the jaws so that it can gently be pulled out. At no time should excessive traction be applied. If the birth canal is particularly dry, then large quantities of obstetrical lubricant should be

inserted via an extension tube – again, only after observing hygienic precautions.
8. Even where gloves have been worn, hands and arms should be thoroughly washed in soap and water following interference.

Surgery
Caesarean section can be performed in the sow but, as an abdominally invasive technique, it can only be done by a veterinary surgeon. Anaesthesia in the field is difficult; access is by a flank incision and antibiotic cover is essential. For the 'pet' pig, the technique is fundamentally the same as that used in the dog.

In most commercial situations, Caesarean section is not economically viable and, where the sow cannot be farrowed, the litter can be retrieved by shooting the sow and cutting out piglets within four minutes. This so-called 'smash and grab' technique is a crude adaptation of that used for hysterectomy rederivation of high-health pigs within a breeding company. It is only viable if early action is taken and a foster sow is available to take the litter.

In conclusion, the farrowing process is a critical period in the breeding life of the sow. In the farming environment, or even with the pet pig, it is the role of the stockman to monitor and assist the sow in achieving a satisfactory outcome – the birth of a litter of live pigs.

CHAPTER THREE

The Perinatal and Neonatal Period

Having successfully negotiated the farrowing process, the next stage is for the baby piglet to become established on the sow. As it will have been born into an environment that is likely to be in the order of 20°C (36°F) cooler than that from which it has come, the first priority for the newborn piglet is to find food and warmth. In order to achieve this, it must negotiate the challenge of being close to a mother that is 200 times its size.

The baby piglet lacks brown fat, has very limited white fat reserves and equally has limited glycogen reserves in the liver and musculature. It is thus critical that the piglet tops up its energy reserves as soon as possible. Moreover, as there is no placental transfer of antibodies from mother to offspring, the piglet is born with minimal immunity against infection. An early suck of colostrum is therefore vital; to provide both food and passive protection, each piglet should obtain a minimum of 75ml (3fl oz) of colostrum in the first six hours of life.

CAUSES OF DEATH IN NEWBORN PIGLETS

Chilling (Hypothermia)

At birth, the piglet has a high surface area to volume ratio, has little insulation and is wet. The immediate effect of the drying process is a drop in body temperature as a result of loss of latent heat through vaporization. In the absence of sufficient energy resources (either

---

Classification of Neonatal Mortality

The commonly recognized causes of death in young piglets are as follows:

- Stillbirth – *see* page 30.
- Overlaying/crushing – *see* page 31.
- Non-viable pigs – *see* page 32.
- Starvation.
- Chilling (hypothermia) – *see* page 29.
- Scour – *see* page 52.
- Meningitis – *see* pages 86 and 101.
- Septicaemia – *see* page 135.
- Savaging.

In most farm situations, the vast majority of deaths are categorized as stillbirth, non-viable or overlaid, although such records can often hide the true cause or causes.

---

internal, such as fat and glycogen, or external, in the form of colostrum), it will be impossible for the piglet to restore this lost heat and its core temperature will consequently continue to fall. The hypothermic animal will initially continue to struggle to seek food and warmth from its mother, thus bringing it into a high-risk area. Additionally, it will become more and more sluggish and will eventually lie down and die 'in its sleep' – unless it is crushed first by the sow. Figure 18 shows the result of hypothermia on subsequent survivability and highlights the need to minimize heat loss.

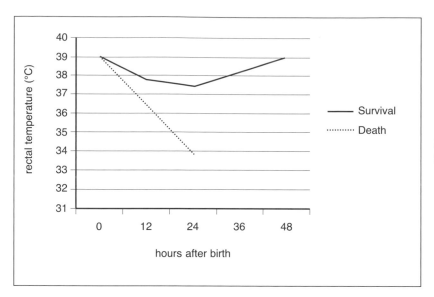

Fig. 18 Changes in body temperature after birth.

Prevention

There are several management techniques that can be employed to minimize the effects of hypothermia:

1. Increase glycogen reserves at birth by increasing the feed level of the sow from thirteen weeks gestation (called 'steaming up').
2. Supervise farrowing – either by employing sufficient staff or by inducing farrowing to control timing.
3. Dry off piglets immediately after birth with paper towels.
4. Use infra-red heat lamps within farrowing crates.
5. Box pigs away under a lamp during the farrowing process.
6. Ensure early and adequate intake of colostrum by supervised and assisted suckling, split or shift suckling, or active dosing of stored colostrum. (Sow colostrum can be expressed from the udder and stored in a deep freeze in 20ml/1fl oz aliquots. Note that it must not be defrosted in a microwave oven.)
7. Provide enclosed creep areas with heating.
8. Provide supplementary energy sources (for example, glucose solution) for small or compromised pigs.

Stillbirths

We have already seen in Chapter 2 that delay in the farrowing process can result in the death of subsequently born pigs. This is a direct result of foetal anoxia. Studies show that, on most farms, 95 per cent of pigs that are truly born dead die at this time, with the remainder dying earlier but not early enough in gestation to have become mummified. However, it is quite possible that some pigs are born alive but are damaged by partial anoxia, or that they become trapped in placental tissue and die rapidly.

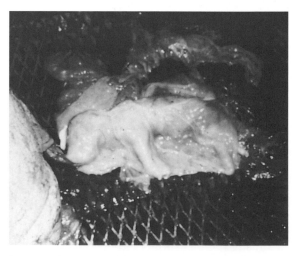

Fig. 19 A single stillborn pig within the placenta.

In reality, when considering strategies to reduce stillbirths such distinctions are of no consequence – the key to reducing death at or around farrowing lies in reducing anoxia by avoiding delays in farrowing. Correct environmental conditions and supervision are crucial in this respect.

An active policy of classifying all early deaths as stillbirths (and thus making mortality figures look better) is misleading. A stillborn pig will have the following features:

1. It will be lying immediately behind the sow, if she is confined.
2. There may be mucus blocking the nostrils and mouth.
3. The claws will contain 'slippers' – soft curved horn.
4. It may be covered in meconium – foetal faeces.

5. Internally, there may be meconium present in the trachea (windpipe) as a result of inhalation of fluid prior to birth.
6. The definitive test of whether a pig was alive at birth is whether the lungs were inflated. If it was alive, a section of lung tissue will float in water; if not, it will sink.

Overlaying/Crushing

Blaming the sow for crushing a piglet to death is often used as a cause of death, although again it sometimes hides the true reasons. Studies on farm have consistently shown that up to 50 per cent of pigs that are crushed to death bear no evidence of having sucked milk or colostrum. In these cases, the true underlying cause of death is starvation and/or chilling, with crushing being the end point. That said, the size discrepancy between mother and offspring means that there is always a risk of

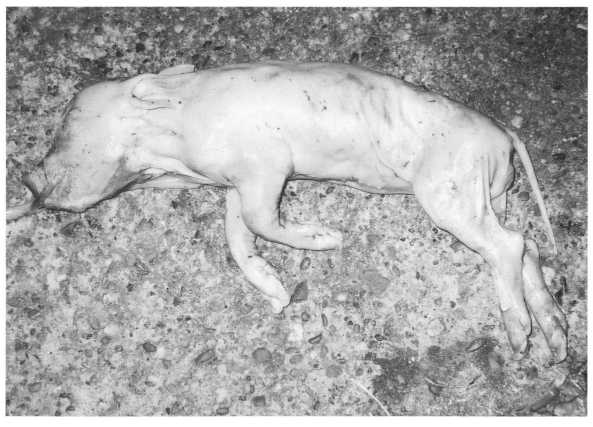

Fig. 20 A stillborn piglet showing slippers on its front feet.

overlaying, which includes literally lying on top of the piglet, standing on the piglet, and trapping the piglet against a bar or wall. In the latter two cases, death may not be instant and the piglet may crawl away to die later – physical injury may not always be obvious.

Prevention
In indoor situations, use of farrowing crates and rails over the years has consistently been shown to cut the incidence of overlaying and remains the most satisfactory arrangement for commercial pig-keeping. In the smallholder and pet-pig situation, supervision of farrowing will overcome the risks associated with stillbirth, chilling, starvation and overlaying.

Non-Viable Pigs

Again, there is a great danger in using this categorization as an excuse for piglet mortality. It literally meaning 'non-liveable', so holds no more meaning than 'the pig was born to die'. There are, however, many situations where this is true, including severe fatal anoxia (*see* 'Stillbirth' above), fatal congenital abnormalities (*see* below) and excessively small piglets.

Studies have shown that, in the modern commercial breeds, a birth weight of 500g (18oz) or less is associated with a very low chance of survival, the piglet's viability increasing in direct proportion to bodyweight at birth. A typical farm would expect birth weights to average around 1.3kg (2lb 14oz) within the range of 400–2,000g (14–70oz); above the higher weight, foetal dystocia as a result of oversize is a risk – *see* page 25. Factors affecting piglet size are listed below:

1. Litter size.
2. Nutrition in early pregnancy with regards placental growth.
3. Nutrition in late pregnancy with regards steaming up.
4. Genetics and breed type.
5. Age of sow – older sows produce more variable piglets, while gilts produce smaller piglets.
6. Health challenge during gestation.

OPPOSITE PAGE:
TOP: *Fig. 21 Arthrogryposis – contraction of flexor tendons.*

BOTTOM LEFT: *Fig. 22 Hydrocephalus – a fluid-filled brain 'cyst' (collapsed following rupture).*

BOTTOM RIGHT: *Fig. 23 Congenital thick forelegs.*

CONGENITAL ABNORMALITIES

Abnormalities present at birth are referred to as congenital. They can arise as a result of a wide range of problems:

1. Genetic mutation in the individual – for example, schistosoma reflexus (*see* Fig. 14), arthrogryposis (*see* Fig. 21) and hydrocephalus (*see* Fig. 22).
2. Inherited defects such as thick forelegs (*see* Fig. 23).
3. Chemical toxicity during pregnancy – for example, particular forms of congenital tremor (*see* page 36).
4. Infectious challenge during pregnancy – for example, classical swine fever, producing congenital tremor (*see* page 36).
5. Nutritional deficiency – for example, vitamin A deficiency, resulting in microphthalmia (small eyes).

Congenital abnormalities tend to occur in a range of circumstances:

1. As sporadic occurrences over long periods of time – particularly true of genetic mutation.
2. As a sudden widespread outbreak – particularly in the case of infectious or toxic insult.
3. As an ongoing low-level problem – particularly with inherited defects such as inguinal hernias.

Figure 24 lists the most common congenital abnormalities seen in the pig and their likely effect on survivability. It should be noted that, in many pigs, multiple abnormalities may occur (for example, cleft palate with hydrocephalus).

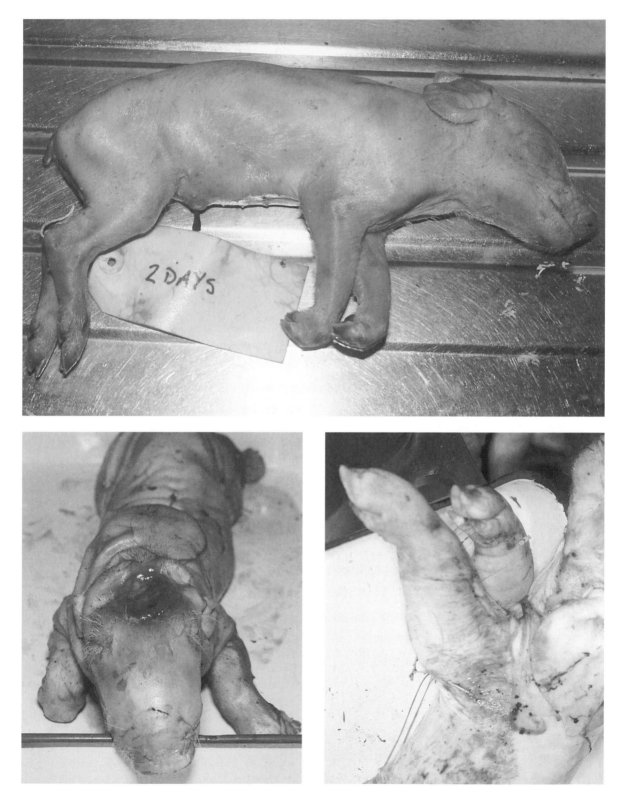

Abnormality	Outcome
Splay-leg	Variable – depends on stockmanship
Congenital tremor	Variable – depends on stockmanship
Hernias/Ruptures	Occasionally fatal later in life. May compromise suitability for slaughter
Kinky tail	No consequence
Thick forelegs	Often fatal
Arthrogryposis	Fatal
Conjoined twins	Fatal
Schistosoma reflexus	Fatal
Cleft Palate	Fatal
Hydrocephalus	Fatal
Epitheliogenesis imperfecta	Survivable if not too severe
Dermatosis vegetans	Fatal
Atresia ani	Fatal in boars. Gilts often survive
Hermaphroditism	No consequence/non-breeding
Microphthalmia	Fatal

Fig. 24 Common congenital abnormalities and their likely effect on survivability.

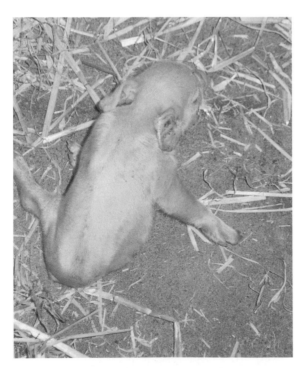

Fig. 25 Hind-leg splay.

Splay-Leg

Splay-leg is probably the most common serious congenital abnormality seen in commercial pig production. At birth, the piglet is unable to keep its legs together, with the result that they splay out sideways. The condition is seen in three distinct forms: hind legs only affected, which is the most common manifestation (*see* Fig. 25); all four legs affected, producing the so-called 'star' (*see* Fig. 26); front legs only affected (extremely rare).

A number of factors can lead to congenital splay-legs:

1. Infection. Damage occurring to the foetus *in utero* can lead to loss of adductor muscle control and splay-leg. PRRS virus can produce a high level of splay-legged pigs and, in particular, is associated with 'stars' and front-leg splays. In addition, any *in utero* challenge to the foetus, if it survives, can lead to muscle weakness that will tend to allow the legs to splay out. This is more the

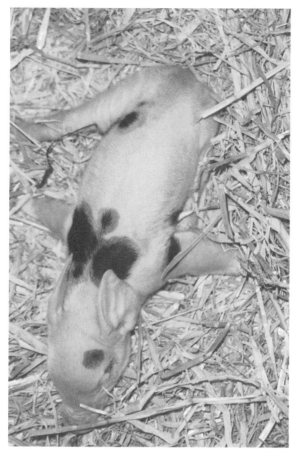

Fig. 26 A piglet splayed on all four legs (a 'star').

case with hind legs, which tend to 'slip' outwards during sucking behaviour.

2. Inherited factors. The Landrace breed is commonly implicated as being more prone to splay-leg than other breed types. Outbreaks of both hind-leg and four-legged splays have been associated with breeding programmes involving high levels of Landrace blood, and there may be familiar trends.

3. Nutrition. Selenium/vitamin E deficiency has been implicated in some cases of splay-leg.

4. Toxicity. Specifically associated with zearalenone (mycotoxin) poisoning, in which four-legged splays occur as a dramatic outbreak.

5. Environment. Probably the most significant factor in the development of hind-leg splay is the slippery nature of the floor for a wet newborn pig, and some surfaces in particular (for example, wide-gap metal slats) are associated with higher incidences of splay-leg. Whether or not there is any inherent weakness in the muscle at birth, as a general rule muscle tone in the newborn pig is poor and a failure to grip, with the resultant sideways slipping of the feet, can lead to muscle damage, particularly of the gluteal mass and the adductor muscles. Without remedial treatment, recovery may not occur.

6. Simultaneous disease. Splay-legs are a common complication of congenital tremor (*see* below).

The obvious consequence of compromised mobility is the high risk of crushing by the sow. A four-legged splay pig is particularly vulnerable and will be further weakened by an inability to suck properly. The same applies to front-leg splay pigs. Pigs that are splayed only in the hind legs can suck and move around and, if not crushed, can survive, although there is a risk of abrasion to the perineum, lower limbs, tail head and nipples.

Treatment
The survival of four-legged and front-legged splays is poor and euthanasia is recommended in such cases. The two principal methods of treatment therefore only really apply to hind-leg splays:

1. Strapping. This involves tying or hobbling the legs together so that the pig can 'bunny-hop' around and the muscles can repair. Electrical insulating tape is preferred and can be tied either around the hocks (*see* Fig. 27) or around the hip joints, passing under the vulva/anus and in front of the tuber ischiae/hook bones (*see* Fig. 28 on page 36). In both cases, hobbling for two to three days is usually sufficient, but care must be taken that the tape is not too tight or that it obscures the anus or vulva.

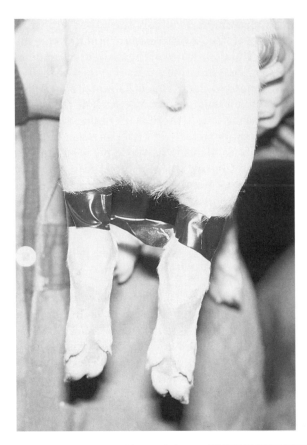

2. Physiotherapy. Vigorous digital massage of the adductor and gluteal muscles for five to ten minutes will often lead to an apparent instant cure; however, pigs may relapse and further massage is needed after a few hours.

As a general rule, splay-leg pigs that survive to forty-eight hours of age have a good chance of recovering and surviving to weaning.

Prevention
Prevention relies upon correcting the trigger factors, controlling disease and, in particular, providing non-slip floors for newborn pigs. Waste carpet can be very usefully employed for this purpose.

Congenital Tremor
Trembling at birth is also referred to as myotonia congenita. There are five distinct recognized causes of the condition, producing varying pathology but all with the same clinical picture:

1. Congenital tremor type AI, resulting from *in utero* infection with the classical swine fever (hog cholera) virus.

ABOVE: *Fig. 27 Hobbling of the hind legs (above the hocks).*

Fig. 28 Repair of splay-leg by tying around the hips (note the tape below the testicles).

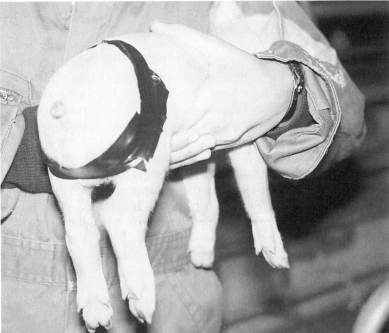

2. Congenital tremor type AII, resulting from unidentified viral infection *in utero* (this is the most common form seen in the field).
3. Congenital tremor type AIII, an inherited condition seen only in male Landrace pigs.
4. Congenital tremor type AIV, an inherited condition occurring in Saddleback progeny as a recessive gene (typically affecting 25 per cent of a litter). There is a variant of type AIV seen in Large White × Saddleback progeny.
5. Congenital tremor type AV, resulting from exposure of the pregnant sow to organophosphates, particularly at around eight to eleven weeks' gestation.

The clinical signs are a variable degree of muscular twitching and trembling, which can be so severe as to prevent sucking. Typically, the trembling ceases when pigs are asleep. Provided pigs are nursed through the condition, they will recover and muscle tremors will usually cease by the time they are weaned. Occasionally, it can take up to eight weeks for trembling to desist.

Prevention and Control
Control and prevention are dependent upon identification of the cause. Where classical swine fever is involved, most developed countries have a slaughter policy. Feedback and acclimatization procedures can be used to control type AII, while alterations to breeding programmes are necessary to control the inherited forms of the disease.

Atresia Ani
The absence of an anus precludes defecation. The piglet will suffer from gradual abdominal distension, condition loss and a slow appearance of jaundice (*see* Fig. 47 on page 59). If the blockage cannot be removed, death will ensue; in such cases, euthanasia is appropriate. In gilts, it is common for a fistula to form between the rectum and the vagina, so that faeces are passed through the vulva. Such animals are clearly unsuitable for breeding purposes but will grow through for slaughter without problem.

Treatment
In cases of simple atresia ani, a cruciate incision where the anus should be is often sufficient to relieve the obstruction permanently. The pig will be faecally incontinent but, in the commercial field, this is unimportant. Unfortunately, however, in the pig the condition is more commonly one of atresia recti, in which the terminal 3–5cm (1–2in) of the rectum is absent rather than there simply being no anus. This is practically inoperable and euthanasia is necessary.

INFECTIOUS DISEASE

The young piglet is vulnerable to a wide range of bacterial and viral infections, producing signs of septicaemia (sudden death), joint ill, diarrhoea and meningitis. Each of these conditions is dealt with in Part 2 of this book, but the key to their control lies in ensuring that hygiene is of a good standard and that colostrum intake is adequate, as described on page 29. As discussed earlier, the influence of hypothermia and colostrum intake are both vital in the immediate post-natal period and are the cause of many problems in the young piglet.

PIGLET PROCESSING

Modern, fast-growing pigs do not obtain sufficient iron from milk to fulfil its requirements for growth and blood formation. Iron-deficiency anaemia can be seen from three weeks of age and can be associated with a low-grade grey diarrhoea; weaning weights with anaemia will be 10 per cent or more below target.

To combat this condition, it is customary to provide iron supplements for piglets, given either orally or by intramuscular injection within the first seven days of life (in the outdoor herd, however, piglets may acquire sufficient iron from the environment and so may not require positive supplementation). Injectable iron is available in the form of iron dextran or in a chelated form as gleptoferron. Iron toxicity can also be seen, particularly when iron dextran has been given to piglets with low vitamin E levels, and can produce sudden death.

SURGICAL INTERVENTION

Tail Docking

Restrictions are in force in certain countries with regards the applicability of tail docking – in the UK, for example, it can only be performed where there is evidence that a failure to dock will lead to problems of tail-biting, while in Norway the procedure is banned altogether. When carried out, tails should be docked within the first three to four days of life and best results can be achieved using some form of thermocautery – either electric- or gas-powered. The amount of tail removed must be sufficient to prevent subsequent biting – on some farms, only the tip needs to be removed, while on others the whole tail must be removed.

Teeth Clipping

The piglet is born with the deciduous corner incisor and canine teeth present, which are needle-sharp. They can therefore do serious damage to other pigs' faces and to the udder of the mothers. Clipping or grinding of the teeth is common practice to avoid oral necrobacillosis (*see* page 119) and mastitis/agalactia (*see* pages 41–2).

Grinding involves the use of a mini angle-grinder; each tooth is ground down close to the gum, either individually or in pairs. This technique is favoured over clipping in some countries – for example, Denmark. More commonly, teeth are clipped using nail- or wire-cutters. The critical point here is to ensure that the teeth are cut close to or flush with the gum, without damaging the latter, and, more critically, that they are not shattered. As the mouth is full of miscellaneous bacteria virtually from birth, these can gain access to the bloodstream if the teeth shatter. If this happens, the most common sequelae is joint ill (*see* page 99). In order to prevent shattering, the clippers should be sharp and one tooth at a time should be clipped. If teeth are clipped in pairs, there is a good chance they will shatter. The technique should be performed early in life but beyond six hours after birth (earlier clipping will inhibit colostrum intake).

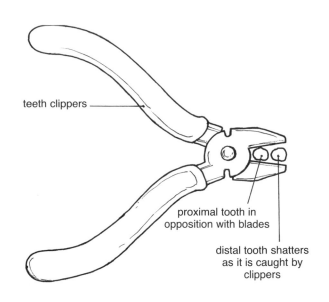

teeth clippers

proximal tooth in opposition with blades

distal tooth shatters as it is caught by clippers

Fig. 29 Teeth clipping.

Castration

Although castration is widely performed, some countries have statutory restrictions on who may castrate, the technique used and the age of pig. In some countries, castration is prohibited. Normally the procedure is carried out within a week of birth without anaesthesia, and an open technique is used. The closed technique can be used by skilled veterinarians on pigs with inguinal hernias but is generally not recommended in the field.

The decision whether or not to castrate will depend largely on the target market for the meat, but it also highlights the tensions that exist between animal welfare, consumer requirements and economic production (castrated males grow slower and less efficiently than their entire counterparts or gilts, and so tend to be fatter).

The period around, and just after, birth is probably the most critical time in a pig's life. In this chapter, we have looked at the major factors compromising viability of the neonate. As with the farrowing process, the stockman can play a huge role in influencing survivability of the piglet.

CHAPTER FOUR

Lactation and Post-Farrowing Problems

The previous chapter discussed the post-natal period from the perspective of the newborn piglet. It is now necessary to address the issues relating to the sow at this time, with particular reference to the factors that compromise milking ability.

LACTATION

Milk production from the developed mammary glands is under hormonal control and coincides with farrowing. The production of milk will gradually increase over the first two weeks of lactation, reaching its peak of 7–9kg (15–20lb) per day by the third week. If the piglets are left to suck, milk will be produced for eight to ten weeks post-farrowing, although the yield declines rapidly beyond six weeks. There is a general perception that the modern lean hybrid sow reaches peak lactation earlier than her ancestors (which possibly reached this point ten to fourteen days post-farrowing) and that the yield declines earlier.

The requirements for a successful lactation are listed below:

1. Mammogenesis.
2. Nutrition (protein and energy).
3. Hormonal control.
4. Stimulation from piglets.
5. Absence of disease
   (both systemic and localized).
6. Body condition.

Initially, the milk is produced in the form of colostrum, which is rich in fat and immunoglobulin (antibodies), but this changes over the first three days to normal milk. The latter will sustain the piglets through to weaning, allowing them to grow at an average of 200g (7oz) per day over twenty-eight days.

Feed and Water Requirements

To stimulate udder development (mammogenesis), sufficient protein (as the building block) and energy (as the fuel) are required. With modern commercial diets, it is usual to keep gilts and sows on low-protein/low-energy diets up until the point of entry to the farrowing area – typically five to seven days prior to farrowing. Such a practice can be associated in gilts with a failure to generate adequate tissue, the result being that the udder is not developed at farrowing and milk/colostrum is not available to the newborn piglets. It may therefore be necessary to switch gilts to a lactator diet (for example, 18 per cent crude protein, 1 per cent lysine) fourteen days before farrowing if such problems occur. This is not usually necessary for sows.

On the day of farrowing, the sow will have little appetite and should be offered low levels of feed. Thereafter, a steady build-up of feed levels is required. Many different feeding regimes have been proposed based on litter size and so on, but as a general principle feed levels should be increased steadily on a daily basis post-farrowing, with no preset upper limit and a target

Day	Morning feed	Evening feed
Day of farrowing	Minimal	Minimal
Day 1	1kg (2lb 3oz)	1kg (2lb 3oz)
Day 2	1kg (2lb 3oz)	1.5kg (3lb 5oz)
Day 3	1.5kg (3lb 5oz)	1.5kg (3lb 5oz)
Day 4	1.5kg (3lb 5oz)	2kg (4lb 6oz)
Day 5	2kg (4lb 6oz)	2kg (4lb 6oz)
Day 6	2kg (4lb 6oz)	2.5kg (5lb 8oz)
Day 7	2.5kg (5lb 8oz)	2.5kg (5lb 8oz)
Day 8	2.5kg (5lb 8oz)	3kg (6lb 10oz)
Day 9	3kg (6lb 10oz)	3kg (6lb 10oz)
Day 10	3kg (6lb 10oz)	3.5kg (7lb 11oz)
Day 11	3.5kg (7lb 11oz)	3.5kg (7lb 11oz)
Day 12	3.5kg (7lb 11oz)	4kg (8lb 13oz)
Day 13	4kg (8lb 13oz)	4kg (8lb 13oz)
Day 14	4kg (8lb 13oz)	4.5kg (9lb 15oz)

Fig. 30 Target feed intake for sows post-farrowing.

of achieving at least three times the maintenance intake. Feed levels should increase by no more than 0.5kg (18oz) dry matter (DM) each day and, with twice-daily feeding, the first increase should be given in the evening feed, when the sow has all night to eat it. A typical feed chart is shown in Figure 30.

It is possible to increase feed intake by up to 10–15 per cent by feeding three times daily, but it is important in such circumstances to ensure a minimum of six hours between each feed (this is the time it takes for the stomach to empty). Always keep in mind that the basic aims of lactation feeding are to maximize milk yield and to minimize weight loss of the sow.

Feed intake will generally be up to 10 per cent higher if it is delivered wet (the feed to water ratio should be between 1:3 and 1:4), but intakes can be boosted on dry feed by adding water on top of the feed when it is offered. If this is carried out regularly, sows will learn to wait for water to be added to feed before eating.

Water requirements for sows increase dramatically during lactation, with 20 litres (4.4 gallons) per day being common. Water-supply systems must, therefore, be designed to fulfil these requirements – flow rates of 1.5 litres (2.6 pints) per minute through nipple drinkers are necessary. It can be argued that flow rates greater than this are needed, but in practice the pressure required to deliver these causes considerable wastage as well as difficulties for the sow to drink.

Other Factors Limiting Milk Yield
In addition to a lack of water and feed, a number of other factors will limit milk yield:

1. High environmental temperatures. Aim for 21°C (70°F) at farrowing, reducing this to 19°C (66°F) after three days (these temperatures should be adjusted to cope with open creep areas and draughts).
2. Stress. Cramped conditions impose a stress on the sow, which limits appetite. This is particularly an issue with large sows in farrowing crates that are too small.
3. Fat mobilization. While the ruminant condition of ketosis/acetonaemia is rarely seen overtly clinically in the sow, farrowing in

excessively fat condition will lead to massive fat mobilization, fat infiltration of the liver and ketone formation. This has a depressive effect on appetite and creates a vicious cycle of inappetance, stimulating further fat mobilization.

4. Stalling. Where feed intake is increased too rapidly post-farrowing, the sow may stall, or refuse feed. The degree to which this happens will largely depend on the genotype of the sow, and feed-level increases must be adjusted accordingly to cope with the circumstances. Ensuring water is freely accessible will go a long way towards avoiding stalling.

5. Disease. *See* below.

POST-FARROWING PROBLEMS IN THE SOW

Mastitis/Metritis/Agalactia (MMA), or Farrowing Fever

The most common disease of the sow around farrowing is usually referred to as MMA or farrowing fever. This is, however, a complex of conditions that may involve infection. The normal temperature of the sow (38.5°C/101.3°F) will rise by up to 1°C (1.8°F) at farrowing time; any increase above this is abnormal and should be investigated.

With MMA the sow will be lethargic, inappetant and reluctant to rise, although often the first sign noticed is dehydration and fading of the litter. Constipation has been linked to the development of MMA (possibly associated with absorption of endotoxins from the gut) and certainly may be relevant in modern commercial systems where sows have free access to straw during gestation but none once they enter the farrowing area.

MMA is also often associated with a vulval discharge post-farrowing, which is assumed to signify metritis (infection and inflammation in the uterus). However, a discharge post-farrowing is, in fact, part of the normal 'cleaning' process for the sow in removing debris from the recently pregnant uterus. Provided the discharge is milky (with or without blood-staining) and not foul-smelling, it is normal. Where the discharge is purulent, thick, foul-smelling and often clotted, this represents pathological change, which signifies either severe ascending infection around farrowing or even retention of piglets.

Treatment and Prevention

Where constipation is associated with the condition, feeding well-soaked bran prior to farrowing is an old-fashioned but effective preventative measure. In cases of abnormal vulval discharge, aggressive antimicrobial treatment is essential if the animal is to survive, and in such cases successful rebreeding may be compromised.

Mastitis

True acute mastitis, where bacteria ascend the teat ducts and colonize the lactogenic tissue, is in practice an uncommon condition, but where it does occur it can have serious consequences for the sow and litter. The most common causative organisms are faecal-based environmental contaminants such as *E. coli* and *Klebsiella*. Circumstances where acute mastitis can become a herd problem include poor hygiene conditions around farrowing and use of certain types of wood-based bedding (especially sawdust).

The condition is usually seen within twenty-four hours of farrowing and presents as an inappetant sow that lies on the udder, preventing the piglets from sucking. Breathing rates will be increased, rectal temperatures may exceed 41°C (106°F) and vomiting may occur. The whole udder will be reddened (hyperaemic), hot, hard and painful. The litter will appear wasted and dehydrated as a result of starvation. Failure to act promptly will often result in death of the sow.

Treatment

Treatment includes appropriate antibiotics in conjunction with non-steroidal anti-inflammatory agents. Oxytocin may be used to assist milk drainage and the removal of bacterial toxins from the udder, but it must be accompanied by hand-milking. Even where the sow survives acute mastitis, total loss of milk production is common and a foster sow is needed for the litter.

Chronic Mastitis

Far more common in sows is chronic mastitis, affecting one or more glands. The most common form is actinomycosis, which is caused by localized bacterial infections, often with *Arcanobacterium pyogenes* (previously called *Actinomyces pyogenes*). Outbreaks of actinomycosis appear to be associated exclusively with straw-based accommodation, possibly implicating soil-borne organisms.

Chronic mastitis is usually seen post-weaning as the udder regresses. One or more glands remain hard, swollen and lumpy, and may ulcerate and produce a discharging abscess. The lesion may partially heal (with or without antimicrobial treatment) as the subsequent pregnancy progresses, only to flare up again as tissue regeneration in the udder occurs prior to the next farrowing. These lesions are permanent, can grow to a very large size so that they drag on the floor, and can lead to considerable discomfort.

Treatment

In situations where soil-borne organisms are believed to be the cause of actinomycosis, herd

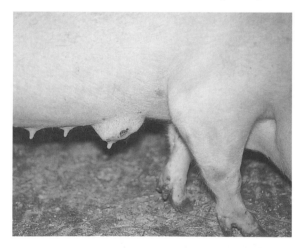

Fig. 31 Mild udder inflammation resulting from Arcanobacterium *(formerly* Actinomyces*) infection.*

medication with tetracyclines may be appropriate. However, in individual cases where large lesions have developed, culling is usually the only option.

Agalactia

A failure to produce milk is termed agalactia, although in practice the term is generally applied to any circumstances where milk supply is compromised. The most common form of agalactia arises as a result of overfeeding the sow prior to farrowing.

If excessive protein and energy are given to the modern high-yielding sow prior to farrowing, then excessive udder development can occur and, in particular, excessive milk is produced in the alveoli. Newborn piglets have a limited milk requirement and the effect of excess production is therefore a build-up of pressure in the udder. This pressure is then exerted on the milk-producing cells that line the alveoli, which initially has a negative-feedback effect on the cells (in other words, they stop producing milk). However, eventually it leads to tissue damage and the release of toxins. At this point, the sow will lose appetite and the udder may become hot and reddened.

The tissue damage created means that as demand from the piglets increases, the udder is no longer able to supply and so the piglets will be seen to 'run off' at seven to ten days of age. This may occur as an individual effect on one or more glands (and hence only one or two pigs may run off), it can affect the whole udder, leading to a complete drying off, or it can simply limit milk production, manifesting as reduced weaning weight in piglets.

In the early stages of the development of this condition, there may be no clinical signs. Where agalactia is seen in herds seven to ten days after farrowing, there is a need to examine sows carefully within twenty-four hours of birth. The whole of the udder should be palpated, particularly at the point where it meets the abdomen, over the whole length on both sides. The mammary tissue should be soft and rounded – like the muscle at the base of one's thumb. Where early stage damage is occurring, this area will

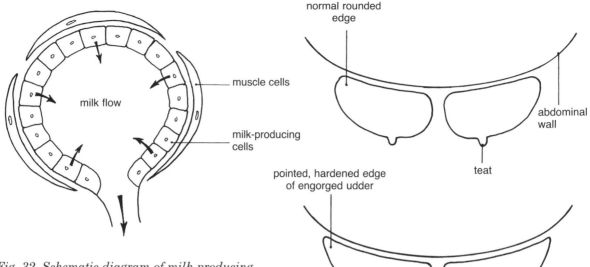

Fig. 32 Schematic diagram of milk-producing alveoli.

Fig. 33 Cross section of udder.

change, becoming hard and more 'pointed', rather like the edge of a finger. If the udder tissue close to the teat is hardened, then the condition is advanced.

Treatment and Prevention
The treatment for this condition is simple and effective, provided it is carried out before serious tissue damage has occurred. The aim is to remove the excess milk before pressure builds up. This can be done in one of two ways:

1. By temporarily adding some older piglets to the sow to 'strip' her out, although care is needed not to spread disease to the young litter, which should be boxed away during this procedure.
2. By hand-milking, assisted by injection of 10IU oxytocin. (Any milk/colostrum collected in this way can be stored in a deep freeze and used as a supplement for other piglets in the future.)

Prevention of the condition is dependent upon avoiding overfeeding in the immediate pre-farrowing period, particularly where high-specification protein-rich diets are used. In particular, feed levels in the period forty-eight hours prior

Gestation day	Feed levels
Up to day 95	2.5kg (5lb 8oz) per day
Days 96–100	3.0kg (6lb 10oz) per day
Days 101–110	3.5kg (7lb 11oz) per day
Days 111–113	2.5kg (5lb 8oz) per day
Days 114–115	1kg (2lb 3oz) per day
Day of farrowing	Minimal

Fig. 34 Suggested feed levels pre-farrowing.

to farrowing should be restricted severely where there is a risk of this condition. A typical feed chart is shown in Figure 34.

Where sows become agitated on very low feed intakes in this pre-farrowing period, they can be offered wet bran as a 'gut filler', which has the added advantage of offsetting the risks of constipation.

Other Causes of Agalactia

Aside from overfeeding, there are several other possible reasons for milk supply problems:

1. Teat damage. Abrasion of the teats may render them 'blind' (in other words, blocked) to the newborn piglet, a condition that will be seen only when the pig farrows for the first time. The front three pairs of teats are most likely to be affected and, where this occurs, protection of them at birth with sticking plaster or solvent-free adhesive is necessary. Torn and otherwise damaged teats in sows may have a similar effect and usually result either from trampling or trapping in slatted floors in a previous lactation. Likewise, inverted nipples may be seen in gilts. These may be of genetic origin and are either blocked, preventing milk release, or are such that piglets cannot suck properly and pressure build-up results.

2. Piglet damage. The needle-sharp teeth of the newborn piglet can cause considerable damage to the teats and udder of the dam. Although true mastitis can result in extreme cases, more commonly there will be a reluctance to suckle, with the sow lying on the udder. This is particularly seen in gilts. Clipping of the teeth will prevent the problem (*see* Chapter 3).

3. Ergot poisoning. Ergot is a fungal toxin (mycotoxin) that reduces blood flow to the extremities and, in severe cases, causes dry gangrene of the limbs, ears, tails and so on. In mild cases in pregnant/farrowed gilts, the reduced blood flow to the udder may prevent tissue generation and milk supply. Avoiding access to mouldy feed or bedding will prevent such problems.

4. Udder oedema. Accumulation of fluid under the skin of the udder is referred to as oedema and is usually seen in large, heavy conditioned sows. When the udder is pressed with the thumb, an impression will be left that will disappear over two to three minutes. The condition is more common in pure-bred animals, particularly the Large White. It is rarely seen outdoors and is probably less common while sows are loose housed during pregnancy. Severe oedema is associated with lack of milk let-down and piglet starvation. Avoidance of excessive body condition is needed to prevent the development of udder oedema; once it has formed, exercise may help reduce the swelling.

5. Adrenalin release. Milk is 'let down' from the udder under the influence of the hormone oxytocin, released from the brain. However, adrenalin is directly antagonistic to the effect of oxytocin, and so where sows or gilts are excitable, milk let-down may be compromised. This is particularly seen in gilts entering farrowing crates for the first time, and in such cases can be offset by ensuring that they are crated five days before farrowing is due. Quiet and gentle handling of sows in the farrowing area is also needed to minimize adrenalin release. The use of music is common in farrowing areas to 'calm' sows and disguise sudden noises. It is of unproven value and should certainly not be so loud that it interferes with the normal vocal communication between sow and litter.

6. Systemic disease. Any systemic illness of the sow may compromise milk production. This is particularly evident in acute PRRS and swine influenza outbreaks (*see* pages 79 and 80), but can occur in any disease situation affecting sows around farrowing and in early lactation.

7. Piglet stimulation. The stimuli for milk production is sucking by piglets. Where piglet health is compromised (for example, through scour, chilling, PRRS and so on), the stimuli will be reduced and so the sow may 'dry up'. In cases of PRRS, it can be difficult to elucidate whether milk failure is the result of the lack of piglet stimulation due to weakened pigs or a direct systemic effect on the dam.

Having successfully negotiated the birth process, the young piglet needs to feed and grow. In this chapter, the importance of lactation has been highlighted, along with the most common factors affecting milk production.

CHAPTER FIVE

Reproductive Diseases of the Boar

As artificial insemination (AI) usage on pig farms increased over the latter part of the twentieth century, the presence of boars on farm declined and, with it, problems specific to the boar. It is not the aim here to discuss details of AI usage or to give an assessment of the influences that affect semen quantity and quality, suffice it to say that the latter is affected by a wide range of factors, including the following:

1. Age.
2. Breed type.
3. Individual variation.
4. Frequency of use.
5. Environmental temperature.
6. Mycotoxins.
7. Nutrition.
8. Systemic disease (*see* page 49).

It is also worth highlighting the fact that, while use of AI cuts down on venereal spread of environmental contaminants, there is a wide range of agents that are capable of being excreted in semen and that may infect the female at insemination. These include:

1. *Leptospira* spp.
2. *Brucella suis*.
3. *Chlamydophora*.
4. Porcine parvovirus.
5. Porcine reproductive and respiratory syndrome (PRRS) virus.
6. Aujeszky's disease virus.
7. Inclusion body rhinitis virus.
8. Classical swine fever virus.
9. Foot and mouth disease virus.
10. Post-weaning multisystemic wasting syndrome (PMWS)/porcine circovirus.

It will be seen that most of the agents listed above are viruses. *Leptospira* spp. are bacteria and are generally controlled by the inclusion of antimicrobial agents in semen diluents.

ANATOMY AND ASSOCIATED PROBLEMS

Sperm are produced in the testes, which are positioned 'outside' the body in such a way that they operate at a temperature 1–2°C (2–4°F) below body temperature. From the testes, sperm are passed into the epididymis for maturation. Fluid is added by the accessory sex glands – of which the paired bulbo-urethral glands are most important in the boar – to produce a large-volume ejaculate (200–500ml/ 7–17fl oz).

The penis, which contains the urethra, lies against the ventral abdomen and has a sigmoid (S-shaped) flexure in front of the scrotum. Erection and protrusion of the penis is achieved through the straightening of this flexure as blood flow to the penis increases pressure. The penis does not increase in size substantially during erection as in the stallion and man. The

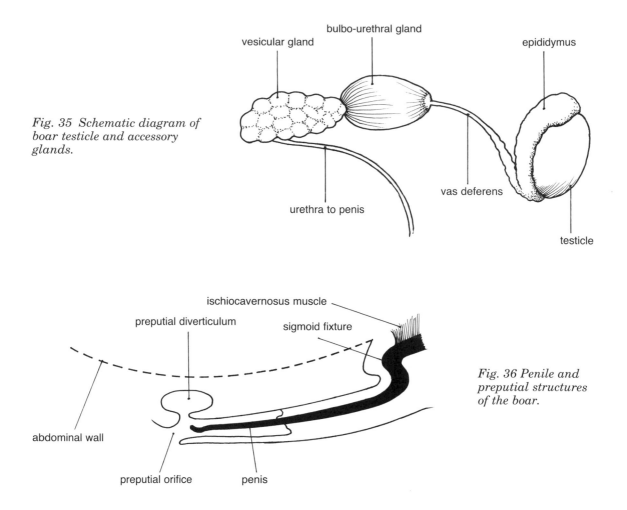

Fig. 35 Schematic diagram of boar testicle and accessory glands.

Fig. 36 Penile and preputial structures of the boar.

tip of the penis has a characteristic corkscrew of three-and-a-half to four turns, which becomes more accentuated during erection and locks into the cervix of the sow at service.

Just inside the preputial orifice between the penis and the body wall is a pouch called the preputial diverticulum, which may have a pheromonal function but is usually filled with a putrid-smelling liquid that is a mixture of urine and decaying semen. This pouch is implicated in some of the clinical problems seen in the boar (*see* Fig. 36).

Erection/Penile Protrusion Failure

Failure of erection in the boar is relatively rare. In the bull, a blood supply bypass system

is well described, in which blood pumped into the penis 'leaks' back out, preventing turgidity. Such a condition may occur in the boar but is extremely rare. Failure of protrusion of the penis occurs as a result of one of the following:

1. Entrapment in the preputial diverticulum, which can easily be manipulated free.
2. Persistence of the frenulum in the young boar, which can cause the penis end to be reflected, thus obstructing protrusion. Even though it is possible to exteriorize the penis manually, the boar will be unable to lock into the cervix and, thus, will be impotent. Surgical resection is possible if the animal is particularly valuable.

3. Adhesions to the prepuce secondary to trauma (*see* below).
4. Constriction of the preputial orifice, either as a congenital abnormality or secondary to trauma.

Blood at Service

The presence of blood on the sheath of the boar or on the sow around or following service is not uncommon but, to understand its significance, it is necessary to work out where it has arisen. The flow chart in Figure 38 should assist in this respect.

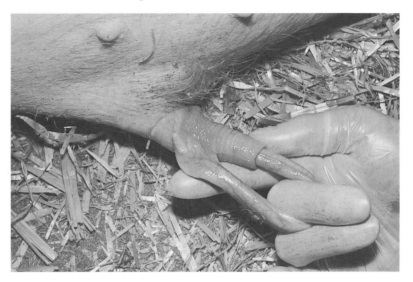

Fig. 37 Persistent frenulum in the penis, causing permanent impotence.

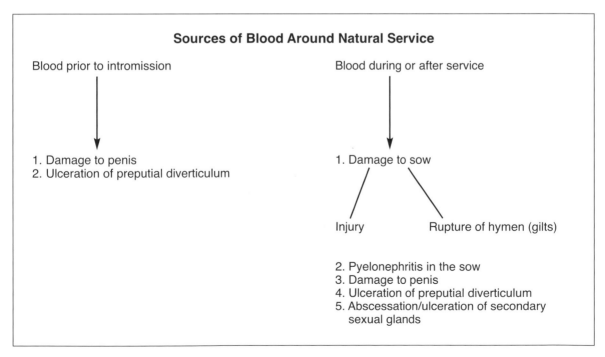

Sources of Blood Around Natural Service

Blood prior to intromission

1. Damage to penis
2. Ulceration of preputial diverticulum

Blood during or after service

1. Damage to sow

Injury   Rupture of hymen (gilts)

2. Pyelonephritis in the sow
3. Damage to penis
4. Ulceration of preputial diverticulum
5. Abscessation/ulceration of secondary sexual glands

Fig. 38

The first aim must be to distinguish between the sow and boar as to which is the source of blood. This is not always easy, although following gilt service small amounts of blood are most likely to come from her rather than the boar. The presence of blood following several matings involving different sows tends to point towards the boar as the source.

It is also necessary to consider the significance of any blood present. Blood, in itself, is not spermicidal and small amounts are of no consequence to fertility. However, if the source is a severely damaged penis, this may not have locked into the sow properly and, thus, mating will have been unsatisfactory. Similarly, if the boar has seriously damaged the sow during mating, it is unlikely that ejaculation will have occurred into the cervix. If the blood arises as a result of infection and ulceration higher up the reproductive tract (accessory glands or testicles), semen quality is likely to be compromised and risks infecting the sow.

INJURY AND DISEASE

Penile Injury
Injuries to the penis are not uncommon and result from trampling or biting by sows/gilts. (They are frequently seen in yarded finishing boars that continually mount one another.)

Treatment
Many such injuries will heal naturally if rested and treated with antimicrobials, but problems can arise with adhesions to the prepuce, which limit future erection and protrusion of the penis. Use of sedatives such as azaperone in boars can lead to prolapse or persistent protrusions of the penis and subsequent damage. Great care is therefore needed in the use of such medication in working boars. Occasionally, damage can be so severe that necrosis of the terminal part of the penis occurs, and some boars may even haemorrhage to death.

Preputial Diverticulum Ulceration
The preputial diverticulum has an uncertain purpose. It may be part of the pheromonal system but some maintain that it is vestigial and is simply a reservoir of putrid and infected fluid. Many stockmen will actively empty the pouch prior to service or semen collection. In the author's experience, ulceration of the diverticulum is common in adult boars, with severe ulcers appearing as buttons that can be felt when the little finger is inserted into the preputial orifice (after the boar has been suitably restrained). The cause of this ulceration is presumed to be the wide range of bacteria present in the pouch, coupled with the chemical effects of the urine and decaying semen found there.

Treatment
Treatment with topical antibiotics (intramammary tubes are suitable) may control infection and allow healing of ulcers where haemorrhage occurs. Complete healing is difficult to achieve and relapse is frequently seen.

Accessory Gland Disease
This is presumed to be the reason behind the presence of blood in the actual ejaculate. Causes of the disease are uncertain, but *Chlamydophora* bacteria have been specifically implicated in the development of such lesions and infection probably ascends from the penis/urethra.

Treatment
When accessory gland disease is diagnosed, treatment involves aggressive broad-spectrum

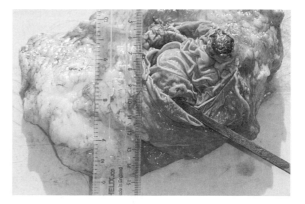

Fig. 39 Ulceration of the preputial diverticulum.

antimicrobial use and a rest period of four to six weeks. In an adult boar, with suitable restraint, it is possible to palpate the bulbo-urethral and vesicular glands via the rectum and, where inflammation is present, pain will be evinced by gentle handling. Great care is needed.

Orchitis

Infection and inflammation of the testicles can result either from injury (for example, biting wounds) or as a result of specific infections such as *Brucella suis*, *Chlamydophora* (chlamydia), blue eye disease and Japanese B encephalitis. The testicles of the boar are frequently asymmetrical and one may be up to 25 per cent longer than the other without any pathological change. However, when affected with orchitis, the testicle will be tense to hard, hot and painful, and visibly swollen. It must be assumed that boars with orchitis are both non-fertile and a source of infection. A consequence of orchitis, if treatable, is atrophy of the testis and total loss of function. If this affects only one testicle, then normal use can be resumed.

Treatment

Antimicrobials are appropriate to treat localized infection and chlamydia infection. In the case of the other listed specific causes, orchitis in the boar is only likely to be one of many signs seen on the farm and whole herd control programmes are needed.

Systemic Disease

As discussed above, testicular function is optimal at a temperature 1–2°C (2–4°F) below body temperature. Where pyrexia occurs, spermatogenesis will therefore be interrupted. Given that it takes between six and eight weeks for full sperm development to occur, it is likely that, following severe systemic disease or heatstroke where body temperature exceeds 41°C (106°F), the boar will be rendered sub-fertile or even sterile for this period. Common diseases where this occurs are erysipelas and *Actinobacillus* pleuropneumonia. Systemic viral disease (for example, classical swine fever) will have similar effects.

There is circumstantial evidence to suggest that boars infected with the PRRS virus may be sub-fertile. If this is the case, the condition is more likely to be a direct effect of the disease rather than as a result of pyrexia, except where the uncommon but severe 'hot' US strains of the virus are involved.

Posthitis/Cellulitis

Oedema (fluid swelling) around the prepuce (*see* Fig. 40) as a result of penetrating subcutaneous infection is a recognized condition. In the

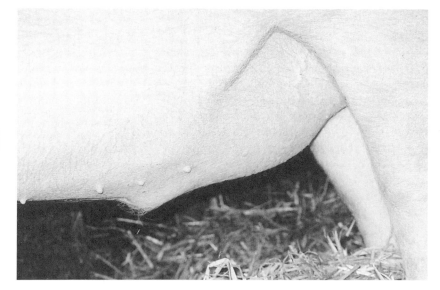

Fig. 40 Posthitis/cellulitis – notice the swelling behind the preputial orifice.

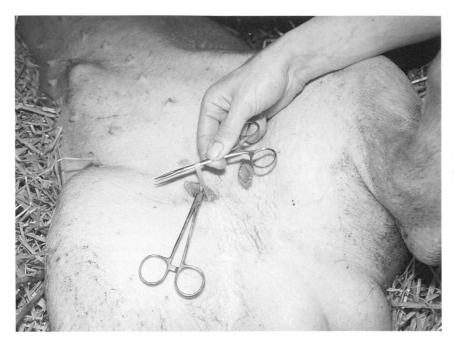

Fig. 41 Exteriorization prior to excision of the vas deferens as part of a vasectomy operation.

author's experience, it has only been seen in AI boars and may arise as a result of manual interference and handling. Bacteria of faecal origin (for example, *Proteus* spp.) penetrate through ulcers that may be obvious in the preputial diverticulum or microscopic in other areas of the preputial mucosa. This infection sets up a cellulitis that spreads out from the prepuce to affect the ventral abdominal wall, and may spread further to produce a mild peritonitis.

Treatment
The condition does not appear to affect either fertility or working ability and is largely intractable to treatment, although its progress can be forestalled with broad-spectrum antimicrobial treatment administered for at least ten days.

SURGICAL INTERVENTION

Preputial Diverticulum Removal
This may be indicated where intractable ulceration and haemorrhage occurs, and it has also been proposed as a method of controlling the endometritis/discharge syndrome in sows. It is rarely performed.

Vasectomy
Use of teaser boars to stimulate oestrous is widely practised. To avoid unplanned pregnancy, removal of a section of the vas deferens from each testis can be performed. This is a surgical exercise and should be undertaken only by a trained veterinary surgeon.

Epididectomy
Removal of the head of the epididymis in piglets one to three weeks of age has been proposed as an alternative to vasectomy. It is easily performed using sharp sterile scissors following a small stab incision on the dorsal side of the testis. In the author's experience, this is an unreliable technique with a high failure rate – in other words, many boars remain fertile.

It is often said that the boar forms 'half the herd'. With the widespread use of artificial insemination in most pig-producing parts of the world, clinical disease in boars on farm has become less of an issue. However, any compromise to the boar's ability to produce fertile semen or to mate successfully can have a dramatic effect on herd reproduction and, thus, the role of the boar should never be understated.

PART 2: General Diseases

CHAPTER SIX

Enteric Disease

Ailments affecting the gastrointestinal or digestive system of the pig can most easily be catalogued in relation to the age of the pig affected, and this applies probably more so than in any other group of ailments related to body systems. In this chapter, we will look at the most important digestive dysfunctions seen in pigs around the world. However, it must be borne in mind that, while many of the conditions described occur principally in predictable ages (for example, swine dysentery in growing pigs), because we are dealing with biological systems variation is inevitable and, on occasions, specific diseases can appear in other age groups.

Although the principal sign of disease in any pig suffering abnormality in the digestive system will be diarrhoea (scour), other signs include vomiting, constipation and abdominal distention. An outline diagram of the digestive system is shown in Fig. 42.

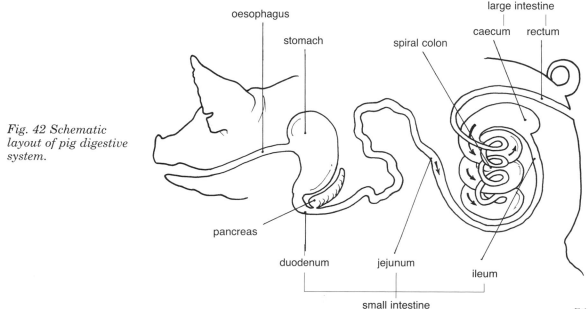

Fig. 42 Schematic layout of pig digestive system.

oesophagus

stomach

large intestine

caecum   rectum

spiral colon

pancreas

duodenum   jejunum

ileum

small intestine

ENTERIC AILMENTS PRIOR TO WEANING

Clostridial Disease

Clostridium perfringens is a soil- and gut-borne bacterium that can cause a range of enteric diseases in the young pig. There are a number of strains that can occur and the nature of the disease will vary with the strain involved. As it is a soil-borne organism, it is always more likely that clostridial disease will be seen in pigs born in outdoor environments, but this does not mean that it does not occur in pigs born indoors. Indeed, in some countries (for example, Denmark) *Clostridium perfringens* is believed to be a major pathogen in indoor pigs. Moreover, a common misconception with regard to the outdoor environment is that clostridia are sheep pathogens, and therefore pasture will present a risk to the pig only if it has previously been grazed by sheep. This is not true. Sheep are particularly vulnerable to clostridial disease and may increase the challenge in a pasture by multiplying the bacteria, but their presence is not necessary for all cases.

The most acute form of clostridial enteritis is caused by *Clostridium perfringens* type C (and very rarely by type B). These strains produce very powerful cytotoxins that damage the gut lining, producing massive haemorrhage (*see* Plate 2). Thus, the principal sign (usually seen within the first few days of life) is the sudden death of whole or part of the litter, with pigs very pale and occasionally with bloody faeces dribbling from the anus. Disease caused by *Clostridium perfringens* type A is much milder, but can be seen from a few hours after birth up to four weeks of age as a low-grade debilitating scour (with a character ranging from watery through to pasty). With this type of infection death is rare.

Treatment

Treatment of pigs and litters infected with any of the strains is extremely difficult owing to toxin production. In cases of type C disease, death may occur so rapidly as to preclude treatment, whereas with type A disease antibiotic therapy gives disappointing results. Support therapy with electrolyte fluid replacement is essential, and the use of penicillin-based oral antibiotics is advisable. However, prevention of disease is far more important.

Prevention and Control

In the short term, disease can be prevented by treating pigs at birth either orally or parentally with a long-acting synthetic penicillin such as amoxycillin. A single dose to all pigs is usually sufficient to prevent type C disease. Type A disease is more difficult to prevent, but a similar approach, possibly combined with treatment of the sow for two to three days prior to birth with similar antibiotics, is sometimes effective.

The long-term control of clostridial disease is best achieved by attention to hygiene and vaccination of the gilt/sow prior to farrowing. A number of sheep vaccines have been cross-licensed for use in the pig, but care must be taken in selecting these to ensure they are aimed at the correct strain. Few cover type A and there is little cross-protection between strains.

E. coli Enteritis

Escherichia coli is another bacterium found ubiquitously in the environment as a result of faecal contamination. *E. coli* are an essential part of the normal gut flora of the pig but there are specific serotypes, such as 0149 (Abotstown), which are enterotoxigenic. All of the pathogenic strains contain adhesins that stick the organism to the wall of the lower small intestine; toxins then released produce a massive fluid outpouring into the gut, which results in an acute watery scour and severe dehydration. Occasionally, the scour is blood-tinged. A key feature of neonatal *E. coli* enteritis is that the pig will continue to suck milk, so that at post-mortem the stomach will contain clotted milk while the small (and/or large) intestine will be distended and filled with gas and fluid.

The source of infection for the neonate is either directly from the mother (the excretion rate of *E. coli* increases in the perinatal period in the sow or gilt) or from a previously contaminated room. Spread of disease will occur from pig to pig and from litter to litter through direct contact with faeces, spread by flies and poor management practices, such as walking from pen to pen and cross-fostering where scour occurs. *E. coli* enteritis can occur at any age in the farrowing house but the most common forms of the disease are seen in the first two or three days of life. However, where disease is seen in older pigs it may be in mixed infection (for example, with rotavirus), or as a *per acute* sudden death, often with a swollen abdomen.

Treatment

Treatment with appropriate antibiotics administered orally is essential, but this must be combined with oral rehydration using electrolyte fluids. It may be necessary to syringe the latter into affected pigs – 20–50ml per hour is the required dose. Provision of warmth and general nursing are also needed to prevent death, either directly from disease or by overlaying as piglets continue to attempt to suckle.

The choice of antibiotic treatment should be based on an antibiogram (sensitivity test), but it should be borne in mind that, over a period of time within a herd, sensitivity patterns will

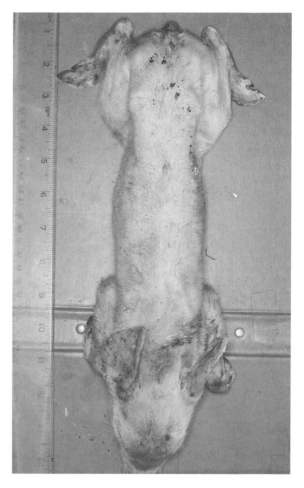

ABOVE: *Fig. 43 Severe dehydration as a result of neonatal* E. coli *infection.*

Fig. 44 A two-day-old piglet with E. coli *infection. Note the inflamed, gas-filled small intestine and empty spiral colon.*

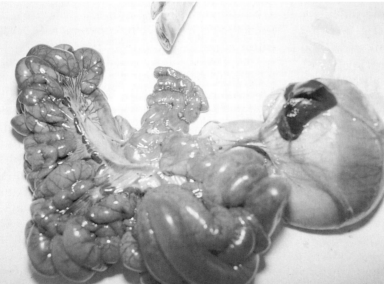

change. *E. coli* belongs to a group of bacteria that can produce transferable antibiotic resistance, so use of any one antibiotic over time will select resistant strains and treatment will fail.

Prevention and Control
In the face of an outbreak of neonatal *E. coli* enteritis, routine preventive antibiotic treatment can be given, preferably orally, at birth. However, this not a long-term solution as resistance will occur rapidly (within three months usually) and disease breakdown will result. Attention to hygiene to reduce the challenge to new litters is therefore vital, and is discussed in detail on page 59.

As with clostridial disease (*see* above), the long-term aim is to promote immunity in the dam that can be transferred to the piglet via colostrum and milk. Given the adhesive property of enterotoxigenic *E. coli*, it is necessary to promote antibodies that bathe the gut lining as opposed to those that are absorbed into the bloodstream. Commercial injectable vaccines promote antibody production in serum, which is then transferred to the colostrum and will bathe the piglets' gut for up to four days. These vaccines will not promote antibodies in milk and, thus, are of value (and are highly effective) only in the neonatal situation. If primary *E. coli* disease occurs above this age, it is necessary to stimulate mucosal immunity additionally using oral vaccination (in other words, feedback – *see* page 60), which is reflected in milk antibody levels.

When administering commercial vaccines, it is preferable to use those with the widest range of antigens and, in particular, those containing the three major adhesins (K88, K99 and 987P) along with the toxins. It should also be mentioned here that antibiotic medication to reduce *E. coli* output from the sow is rarely successful and is ill-advised on the grounds of abuse of medicines and development of resistance.

Rotavirus
Rotaviruses are common organisms found within a pig population, so the presence of such virus does not always mean that they are the cause of the disease. There are a number of strains of rotavirus and, as with *Clostridium perfringens*, there is no cross-protection between strains and it is possible that pigs can suffer sequential disease with different strains.

Scour results from damage to the cellular lining of the small intestine, such that the absorptive villi shrink and reduce the ability of the gut to digest and absorb nutrients. An osmotic scour will result and can range from profusely watery in character to soft, pasty, yellow faeces. Blood is not a feature of rotaviral scour unless infection is complicated by other agents such as coccidia, and primary death is rare – any losses generally result from dehydration or crushing by the sow. Disease may be seen as early as twenty-four hours of age right through to weaning and beyond. Rotaviral scour can be diagnosed only by sophisticated laboratory tests that will distinguish it from other causes.

Treatment
As a viral disease, there is no specific treatment available. It is, however, common for rotavirus disease to occur in conjunction with *E. coli* infection, and treatment here is appropriate. As with all enteric disease in sucking piglets, dehydration is the major problem and so oral rehydration therapy using electrolytes is an essential part of nursing pigs through the illness. Comfort and warmth are also vital. In uncomplicated infection, recovery will occur within three to four days.

Prevention and Control
Prevention of rotaviral scour depends on a combination of reducing challenge (through good hygiene) and ensuring immunity in the mothers that is passed on in colostrum and milk. There are no commercial vaccines available for pigs at present and the cattle rotaviral vaccines contain only one strain of rotavirus, which is one of the least common in the pig. There is also a tendency for this vaccine to be prohibitively expensive for use in the pig. Feedback is the most cost-effective technique available for rotavirus control (*see* page 60).

Coronaviral Diseases

This group of viruses causes some of the most dramatic outbreaks of enteric disease in pigs. Transmissible gastroenteritis (TGE) is the most severe and in most herds tends to behave in an epidemic form, causing a dramatic outbreak of scour in pigs of all ages. The younger the pigs affected, the more severe the outcome, to the extent that pigs less than a week old tend to suffer 100 per cent mortality. In addition to profuse watery diarrhoea, often green in colour, vomiting may be seen in younger piglets. In older pigs, the disease is less severe but even adult pigs can be affected. The key to the diagnosis lies in the pattern of disease, in which all ages are affected.

There is evidence to suggest that non-pathogenic strains of TGE virus now exist, but the decline in the incidence of this disease in many parts of the world has been attributed to a mutation that occurred in the mid-1980s in Europe. This mutation produced porcine respiratory coronavirus, a virtually non-pathogenic respiratory-based virus that spread rapidly through and between herds, and that provides cross-immunity for TGE.

Epidemic diarrhoea (PED) is a similar virus to TEG, although they do not share cross-immunity and PED produces a milder form of the disease. There are two forms of PED, one of which affects only sucking piglets and the other, like TGE, affecting all age groups. Mortality in either case is much lower than with TGE but the diseases are otherwise indistinguishable.

These viruses do damage similar to that caused by rotavirus: the villi of the intestine become shrunken, reducing the ability of the pig to digest and absorb nutrients. Dehydration is often extreme in the youngest pigs. While most outbreaks of TGE and PED tend to be epizootic (in other words, explosive and short-lived in a herd), enzootic disease can occur and may form part of the grower scour picture described on page 63.

Treatment

As with rotavirus, treatment is non-specific and, in the case of very young pigs with TGE, it is probably not justifiable. Electrolytes may provide an aid to recovery in less severe cases, with diarrhoea ceasing two to three days after treatment is commenced. It should be noted that owing to the extremely high mortality with TGE, sows tend to be weaned soon after farrowing. This can have important implications for the future breeding ability of individuals and for the future productivity of a herd. For a discussion on this, *see* Chapter 1.

Prevention and Control

TGE and PED viruses are easily spread by birds, especially starlings, and measures must be taken to prevent ingress and contamination of feed supplies. Obviously, avoidance of introduction of contaminated pigs is a vital biosecurity measure and relies on veterinary liaison and quarantine protocols.

Once an outbreak occurs within a herd, it is essential that its spread throughout is accelerated to allow immunity to build up and, hence, the disease to die down. In particular, it is important that pregnant sows are exposed to the viruses in order to protect their future litter when born, even though this is likely to produce mild disease in them that can occasionally be severe enough to have the secondary effect of causing abortion. Again, feedback is the best approach, although legislation may restrict the ability to spread the disease successfully (*see* page 60).

Vomiting and Wasting Disease (VWD)

This is another coronavirus infection, which affects pigs aged from five days to three weeks, usually as a sporadic disease. It differs from the other viruses described here in that it does not cause diarrhoea (scour). As the name suggests, the principal signs are vomiting and loss of condition, resulting in death, with constipation a notable feature. The disease may affect only part of a litter and is fatal.

Treatment

No treatment for affected pigs is available. The disease is uncommon owing to the high background level of the virus in herds, this producing sows that are mostly immune (although the incidence of serological-positive sows varies widely and, in some countries – for example, Northern Ireland and Japan – is low).

Prevention and Control
Prevention of the disease depends on ensuring that replacement gilts are exposed to the virus prior to breeding. This can be achieved by attention to acclimatization procedures.

Porcine Reproductive and Respiratory Syndrome (PRRS, or Blue Ear Disease)

It may seem strange to include a disease of reproduction and the respiratory system in this section on enteric ailments. However, in a naive herd suffering a breakdown with PRRS, in which all animals can show some signs of disease, the sucking piglet can be affected with a severe intractable and debilitating scour. Such an acute outbreak may last six to eight weeks in a commercial herd, during which time farrowing-house mortality can exceed 50 per cent. Many of these pigs will be born weak and suffer other infections such as joint ill, but scour is a frequent problem.

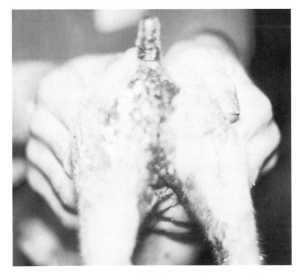

Fig. 45 Severe perineal inflammation resulting from scalding by acute diarrhoea (porcine reproductive and respiratory syndrome infection).

Treatment
As PRRS is a viral disease, specific treatment is not available. Nursing care using electrolytes, milk supplements and antibiotic cover can, however, limit the losses incurred.

Prevention and Control
The prevention and control of PRRS is covered in detail in Chapters 1 and 7.

Coccidiosis

Most food-producing species of animals can be infected with, and affected by, coccidiosis, although in general terms the different coccidia are host-specific. The cause of disease in the pig is *Isospora suis*, which, like *E. coli*, is ubiquitous in pig populations and causes disease only if environmental conditions allow. Within the UK and western Europe, coccidiosis is probably the most common cause of diarrhoea in pigs during the second and third weeks of life.

Isospora suis is a parasitic organism that has a life cycle partially in the pig and partially in the environment. Because of this life cycle, it is not possible for disease to be seen below five days of age and it usually occurs between days ten and fourteen. The scour produced is generally mild, pasty and usually yellow, although it may contain very small blood flecks that can be seen on close examination.

Mortality is rare with piglet coccidiosis but it can have a debilitating effect so as to reduce weaning weights on a herd average by up to 1kg (2lb 3oz) per piglet at twenty-four days. Another key feature of coccidiosis is its poor response to treatment. The damage done – principally to the small intestine – is to render the pig intolerant to milk, thereby preventing its digestion. A typical feature, therefore, is that scour due to coccidiosis ceases at weaning.

Treatment
Treatment of piglets already scouring with coccidiosis is frequently unsuccessful, although specific anti-coccidial agents (for example, toltrazuril) has been tried. Sulphonamide-based treatments, administered either orally or by injection, can also be attempted. As with

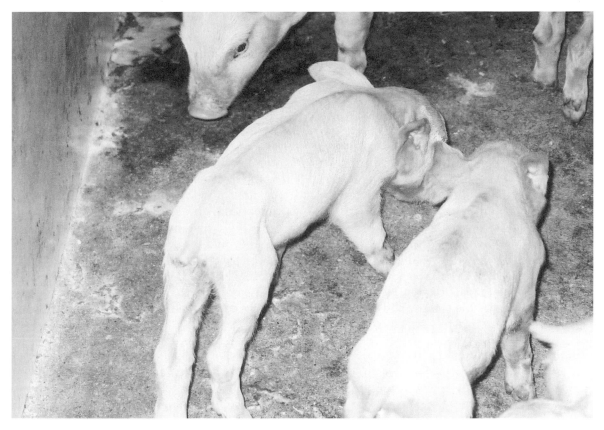

Fig. 46 Yellow pasty scour and loss of condition in ten-day-old piglets typical of coccidiosis.

all scours in piglets, freely available fluids, including electrolytes, are essential as an aid to nursing.

Prevention and Control

The nature of *Isopora suis* is such that contamination of the farrowing pen is the key to development of the disease. The original infection may be seeded by the sow, but it is the carrying over of infection from one litter to the next that perpetuates disease. The infectious particles produced by affected piglets (oocysts) are extremely resistant to drying and disinfection. They undergo a maturing phase in the pen before they are able to reinfest a pig, and thus maturation is temperature-dependent, occurring faster in warm weather. In modern pig-keeping systems, the disease may be seen all year round, but in the outdoor situation it

is rare in winter. Solid-floor farrowing systems, particularly those that are not thoroughly cleaned and correctly disinfected, are particularly at risk of coccidiosis.

The routine use of toltrazuril to prevent coccidiosis is now widespread, although the medication is only licensed for use in pigs in a few countries such as Australia. The drug is widely available elsewhere as a poultry medication, but this formulation is very unpalatable to pigs and can invoke immediate vomiting or regurgitation, although this reaction is highly variable between farms. If a reaction does occur, it is necessary to dilute the drug with water or even glycerol.

Timing of treatment is vital for effective activity – it is necessary to wait long enough for the *Isopora* to develop to a stage that is vulnerable. Provided initial infection occurs within twenty-four hours of birth, the fourth day of life is the most effective time to treat. By killing the developing merozoites at this stage, immunity appears to develop and the pig is protected through to weaning. If pigs occupy a two-stage farrowing/rearing area, the optimum treatment time can occur four days after a move. In very heavily contaminated environments, it may be necessary to treat for a second time at ten days of age. To break the cycle of disease within a farrowing area, it may be necessary to undertake a specific cleaning programme using highly specialized disinfectants (*see* below).

Coccidiosis with various species of *Eimeria* may occur in weaned pigs and growers, but this is rare and it is doubtful whether these are primary pathogens. Cryptosporidiosis is related to coccidiosis in suckling pigs. This disease is very rare, impossible to treat and can be controlled only by strict hygiene measures.

Nutritional Scours

'Nutritional' scours are common in piglets sucking milk from the sow and tend to occur in three situations:

1. Milk overload. As the pig grows towards weaning, the milk intake may simply be too great for the digestive system.
2. Abnormalities in milk. These occur as a result of disease in the sow, unusual ingredients in sow feed and certain hormonal changes taking place in the sow, the milk character altering such that digestibility is affected.
3. Creep feed. It is common practice to provide piglets with hard feed prior to weaning. If this feed is allowed to go stale (rancid) or is taken in excessive amounts, the piglet's digestibility is upset and scour can result.

Prevention and Control

In all these cases, withdrawal of the offending nutrients – either by weaning, restricting access to sucking or removal of creep – will allow rapid resolution. Poor hygiene within a farrowing pen can, however, exacerbate nutritional scours by allowing an overload of the gut with opportunist secondary bacteria and other microbes.

Gut Obstruction

Obstruction of the gut of the young pig can occur in two situations:

1. Atresia ani, where the patency of the anus is not established from birth (in other words, this is a congenital abnormality). In many such cases the terminal rectum may be absent as well. If the condition goes unnoticed, the abdomen will become progressively distended as the piglet becomes weaker and loses condition (*see* Fig. 47). In such cases euthanasia is essential. In gilts, a fistula can form between the rectum (if of sufficient length) and the vagina, such that faeces can still be voided via the vulva. This may not be noticed until the animal reaches breeding age.
2. Ingestion of wood shavings. Where wood shavings are used as bedding, some piglets will ingest them and they can impact in the gut, usually causing a blockage at the ileo-caeco-colic valve (the junction between the small and large intestines). Death will tend to occur rapidly due to toxic shock, and in such cases the impaction will only be noted at post-mortem examination.

Diagnosis of Piglet Enteric Diseases

While the age affected, the severity of disease and the nature of the clinical presentation may enable a provisional diagnosis to be reached, it is vital that a precise diagnosis is made if appropriate long-term control measures are to be put into place. A wide range of complex tests are available for each of the conditions described above, but for practical purposes here we need only concern ourselves with the nature of samples required.

At the simplest level, when suspecting *E. coli* enteritis, dry swabs should be collected from the rectum of several affected, untreated pigs (one swab can be used for up to six pigs) and tested for bacteriology. Growth of pure haemolytic *E. coli* would support a provisional

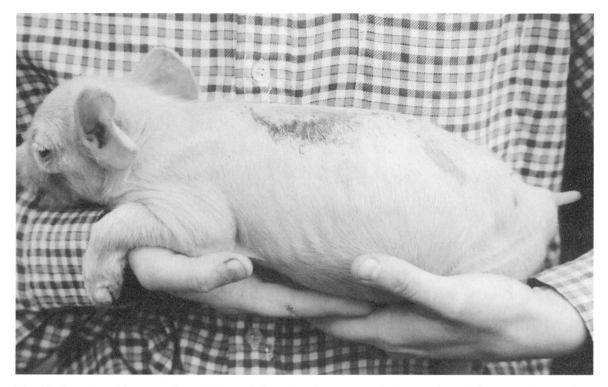

Fig. 47 Atresia ani in a ten-day-old boar piglet. Note the poor condition, swollen abdomen and protruding perineum.

diagnosis and serotyping can follow. Importantly, a quick sensitivity test can be done to assist treatment choice. However, swabs are of no value in diagnosing any of the other conditions, and if a mixed culture of bacteria is grown, this tells little of the cause of infection.

Collection of the actual scour into a sterile pot would allow toxin tests for clostridia and PAGE tests for rotavirus. However, these tests show only whether the organism or its toxin is present; they do not confirm the actual cause of the scour.

Post-mortem examination of new cases of untreated pigs submitted alive to the laboratory or processed on farm will yield the best results. Samples of gut must be fixed in preservative (formal saline) within ten minutes of the pig's death, and can be examined histopathologically (under a microscope) to look for specific tissue damage. Such examination can give a definitive diagnosis, such as in coccidiosis (it is the only way to diagnose this disease reliably), and can support other findings (for example, villous atrophy along with a positive rotavirus test would tend to confirm rotavirus as the cause of the problem). Such an approach is essential if complex infections are involved. Ideally, several pigs should be sacrificed to achieve an accurate diagnosis.

Prevention of Piglet Enteric Diseases

Reducing the infectious challenge and boosting immunity transferred from sow to piglet have been highlighted as the principal measures to control enteric disease in the piglet.

Hygiene

All farrowing areas should operate on an all in/all out basis to facilitate cleaning and to avoid mixing pigs of differing ages within a common area (otherwise, disease would spread from older to younger pigs). In the outdoor

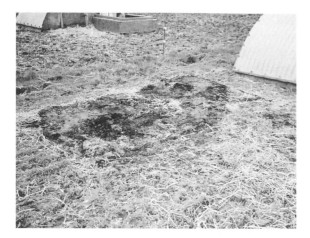

Fig. 48 Burning bedding outdoors is equivalent to power-washing farrowing pens indoors.

environment, this practice relates to the paddock rather than a room.

Following emptying, all solid manure and bedding must be removed and destroyed (outdoors it could be burnt *in situ* if not too wet). Indoor farrowing pens should then be soaked with a detergent. (Both sow lactator diet and piglet creep diets are high in oil, and this tends to produce a film of grease that will protect microbes if it is not broken down.) Power-washing should follow, in which all visible organic material is washed out. Slurry channels should also have been emptied and then washed.

Only once all organic matter is removed should disinfectants be applied – at the measured recommended rate of application. If too dilute, they will not work; if too strong, there will be a waste and possibly a risk of scalding when the area is repopulated. As a final measure, the room should be fumigated, either with formaldehyde/potassium permanganate or with a specific anti-coccidial agent. An alternative, and one that is particularly useful for solid-floor systems, is limewashing. A thick emulsion of hydrated lime is made up and applied to all surfaces, although it must be left to cure for four days to avoid serious skin damage to pigs from the caustic effects of the very high pH.

Outdoors, arcs are simply moved to fresh, clean ground for each cycle of farrowing.

Promoting Immunity

In the absence of suitable commercial vaccines (for example, to treat rotavirus), the only way to stimulate immunity in the sow is to expose her to natural infection, at a time that will not damage her or her unborn litter. This is the procedure known as feedback and, with respect to preventing neonatal scour, is best targeted in the last month of pregnancy. Historically, feedback using gut material from dead affected pigs has been used, as in outbreaks of TGE and PED. However, this is not now permitted in some countries (in the UK, for instance) and faecal material must be relied on solely as a source of infection. The richest source of organisms that cause scour is the scour itself, and this should be collected either with bedding material, wiped up with tissues or collected direct from the pig by compressing the abdomen (gently!) while lifting the tail.

The material should be diluted in equal proportions with clean water and then presented to sows that are more than eighty-five days pregnant twice weekly at a dose rate of 5ml per sow. It is critical that the following rules are applied:

1. Feedback is not given to sows of less than seventy-five days gestation, as incidental viruses can damage developing foetuses below this age.
2. Feedback ceases prior to the sow's entry to the farrowing house – you do not want to introduce disease into a clean building deliberately.
3. Scour from piglets suffering from PRRS is not used in feedback, as this virus will damage the sow and foetuses at any stage of pregnancy.
4. If feedback coincides with any illness in sows, *stop immediately*. Feedback is a very crude form of vaccinating. Unfortunately, it is impossible to know whether feedback material contains what is needed or whether it contains other pathological agents (Erysipelas, for example) that can damage the sow.

ENTERIC DISEASE IN WEANERS

Post-Weaning Scour

Enteritis in piglets aged from three to eight weeks generally falls into the bracket of post-weaning diarrhoea. *E. coli* and *Salmonella* spp. are the most common causative organisms for scour at this stage.

In the modern 'crash' weaning system operated on most commercial pig farms, the piglet digestive system has to cope with a rapid change from a warm liquid diet 'on tap', comprising easily digestible fats, sugars and protein, to a dry pelleted feed. While the latter is often provided ad lib, there is no behavioural stimulus to eat, and the food consists of complex carbohydrates, long-chain proteins and more complex fats. The consequence of this is that when the pelleted food is eaten, particularly if taken in one large meal (gorging), much of it passes through the small intestine in an undigested state and forms a substrate for microbial proliferation. Specific pathogenic strains of *E. coli* can thrive in such conditions (these are usually different strains to those found in the neonatal situation), producing an acute diarrhoea within seven days of weaning. This is frequently fatal. *Salmonella typhimurium* and

Salmonella derby are also capable of producing such disease, and so the microbial causes of post-weaning scour can be unravelled only in a laboratory. (In some cases, *Salmonella* can also produce a severe necrotic enteritis in weaners.)

Treatment
Early and aggressive antimicrobial therapy is needed to treat affected pigs, with the choice of treatment determined or verified using an antibiogram, or sensitivity test. Treatment can be given by injection or, in less severe cases, through water. Free access to water or electrolytes is also essential.

Prevention and Control
Prevention of post-weaning scours relies upon a number of broad principles, as follows:

1. The challenge of microbes to the pig should be minimized by weaning into a spotlessly clean environment (*see* page 59) and through the operation of an all-in/all-out system.
2. Chilling and draughts should be avoided, as these are major triggers for scour. When the pig is chilled, blood flow is withdrawn from non-vital organs, including the gut, which stops contracting. This allows bacterial

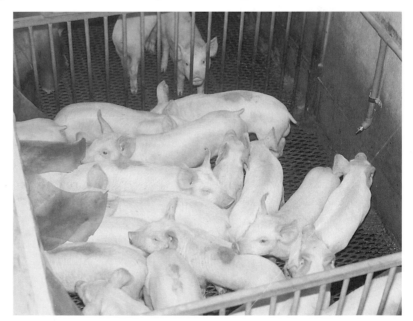

Fig. 49 Loss of condition and scour typical of post-weaning E. coli *enteritis.*

growth without the normal flushing-out effect.

3. Gorging should be prevented by providing food on a little and often basis in troughs that all pigs can access simultaneously. Only the highest quality starter diets should be used, containing animal protein, cooked cereals and light oils such as coconut oil. In some situations, fermented liquid feed has been used post-weaning, but this requires highly specialized equipment and experience.

Preventative medication can be used in a range of forms:

1. By injection, usually only in the severest of outbreaks and as a short-term measure.
2. In water as a strategic treatment prior to the expected problems.
3. In feed, to cover a two-week period. High levels of non-soluble zinc (as zinc oxide) are used throughout Europe and elsewhere as a non-antibiotic control measure, which is highly effective but only if used from weaning. It appears to prevent the growth of bacteria, but will not kill them off once they are present in high numbers.

Vaccination as a method of controlling post-weaning diarrhoea is generally very disappointing.

Post-Weaning Multisystemic Wasting Syndrome (PMWS)

This is a complex disease process that affects the respiratory system (*see* page 83), immune system and skin, and ultimately leads to death in pigs as they suffer a dramatic loss of condition. One of the most common presenting signs is a profuse watery scour in pigs typically five to eight weeks of age, this frequently being of variable colour (green to yellow to brown) and with a pungent aroma. The diarrhoea will pass down the perineum and often cause scalding of the skin. Weight loss will be dramatic.

Control
The control of this disease is dealt with in Chapter 7 (*see* page 83).

Ileitis

Formally known as porcine intestinal adenomatosis (PIA), this disease is caused by a novel intracellular bacteria called *Lawsonia intracellularis*, which studies have shown is

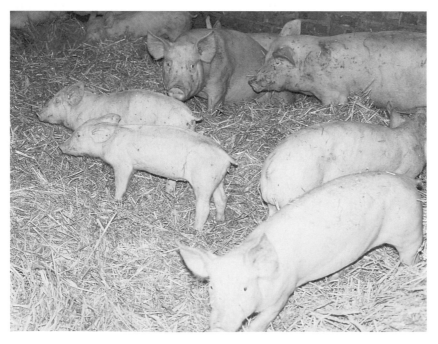

Fig. 50 Severe loss of condition typical of post-weaning multisystemic wasting syndrome (PMWS) with severe scour.

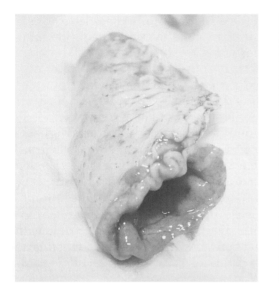

Fig. 51 *Thickening of the ileum as a result of* Lawsonia *infection.*

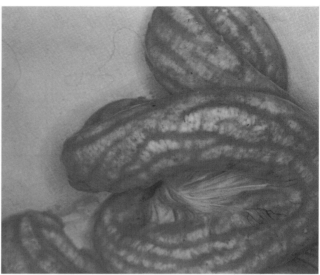

Fig. 52 *Severely thickened hosepipe gut is occasionally seen as part of the porcine intestinal adenomatosis (PIA), or ileitis, complex.*

present in more than 95 per cent of pig farms in western Europe (France, Germany and the UK). It is capable of producing a low-grade grey scour, mainly due to thickening of the intestinal wall, and occurs in pigs from as young as three to four weeks, but typically appears at seven to eight weeks and throughout the growing phase. In extreme conditions, severe thickening of the intestine produces a so-called 'hosepipe' gut. In such cases, recovery is rare.

At the younger end, it can be difficult to differentiate ileitis from PMWS, although it is usually less severe and weight loss is less marked. Generally, mortality is low but growth rates from weaning to slaughter can be depressed by more than 10 per cent. In older pigs, ileitis can be associated with non-specific grower scours (*see* below).

Treatment
The causative organism is extremely sensitive to such antimicrobials as tylosin and tetracyclines, but as an intracellular organism is best treated with an antibiotic that penetrates the cell wall, such as tylosin. Treatment of affected pigs via water is preferable, although

prevention by inclusion of low levels of tylosin in feed (40ppm) can be highly effective. A new generation of vaccines is arriving that will immunize against *Lawsonia* infection. These are unusual in that they are administered orally via the water system and not parentally through a needle and syringe.

Prevention and Control
Once again, hygiene is a key feature in the control of this disease.

ENTERIC DISEASE IN GROWING PIGS

'Colitis'
A group of conditions under the title of colitis has been recognized since the 1980s as a cause of generally low-grade diarrhoea and loss of condition in pigs weighing 20–70kg (45–155lb). Colitis literally means 'inflammation of the colon', but this can be something of a misnomer; the condition seen involves the lower small intestine, either instead of or as well as the colon (the major part of the large intestine). Perhaps 'grower scours' would be a better term.

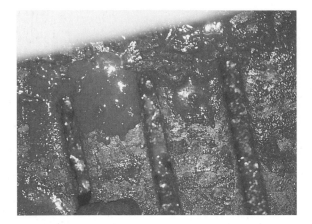

Fig. 53 Grey, watery faeces typical of grower scours or colitis.

Where the colon is affected, the resulting irritation is caused by an increase in mucus production, which is evident in the scour as jelly. Fresh blood flecks may also occur, but in both the inflammation of the colon and small intestine this is a feature only of the more severe forms of the disease. A grey 'cow pat' is a more common indicator.

Grower scours are a complex interaction between nutrition and infection, and, as such, can be controlled by attending to the nutritional needs of the pig and reducing the levels of microbial challenge. In much the same way as post-weaning *E. coli* disease results from the inability of the pig to digest novel feed, which then forms a substrate for microbial proliferation lower down the digestive tract, grower scours may follow a similar pathogenesis. It is widely regarded in the UK that the condition has escalated since dietary copper levels were reduced in early 2004.

Where dry feed is supplied, the cereals (wheat and barley primarily) contain a variable amount of non-starch polysaccharides such as arabinose and xylose. In their natural form, these chemicals are indigestible to the pig and pass straight through the gut untouched. However, if they are heated – as occurs during the pelleting process – they are altered in such a way that each molecule absorbs water. As these

altered molecules pass into the colon, the normal microbial flora attacks them, breaking them down and releasing the water. There are two effects of this. First, the excess water may overload the gut, simply increasing the water content of the faeces. It takes only an increase of 2–3 per cent water content to turn a normal, fully formed stool into a 'cow pat' or worse. Second, the microbes will proliferate and cause direct damage to the gut, altering function and causing diarrhoea.

A wide range of microbes have been implicated in grower scours, including *Brachyspira pilosicoli*, *Yersinia enterocolitica*, *Salmonella* spp. and *Lawsonia intracellularis*. Organisms such as *Eimera* spp. (coccidia) and *Balantidium coli* may also be implicated but these are not primary pathogens, simply opportunists taking advantage of a damaged gut. Overfeeding may also be implicated in the development of grower scours by simply overloading the small intestine. This is a particular feature of pigs weighing 20–25kg (45–55lb) upwards that are starting to eat wet feed. The initial change of diet form upsets digestion and scour frequently results.

Treatment and Control

While short-term antibiotic medication may be needed in feed or water to control a problem, the long-term control lies in nutritional management. Grower scours are less common in meal-fed pigs and in pigs fed restricted diets. However, studies have regularly confirmed that the fastest and most efficient growth is achieved by ad lib feeding of pellets. Research work is needed to identify strains of corn that are less harmful, but at the same time enzymes that break down the non-starch polysaccharides are being developed to include in feed so that the problem can be alleviated. (Studies have shown that feeding cooked white rice minimizes maldigestion and grower scours, but this is hardly an economic option.)

Any feed changes should be gradual, with old and new diets ideally mixed together for up to a week to smooth the transition. When changing from dry to wet feeding, the wet feed should either be supplied ad lib or, preferably, on a little and often basis (four to six feeds per day) until the pigs are used to it.

Swine Dysentery

This is a disease caused by the bacterium *Brachyspira hyodysenteriae*, which in its typical form produces an ulcerative colitis characterized by severe diarrhoea containing blood and mucus, accompanied by a raised temperature, depression and severe loss of condition (*see* Plate 3). Death is not unknown as a primary effect but, probably more significantly, is a result of the debilitating effect of the disease, which opens the door to secondary conditions such as pneumonia. In many endemic situations, swine dysentery is indistinguishable from grower scours and so complex diagnostic methods are needed to unravel the microbial picture.

One of the key features of swine dysentery is its ability to remain a permanent problem within a herd. The organism appears to stay in the environment or be permanently excreted by recovered pigs, which thereby act as a source of infection for vulnerable progeny following through the farm in a continual-flow set-up such as a breeder-feeder farm. While the typical presentation of the disease is in growing pigs ten to twenty weeks old, it can occur in a primary breakdown situation in sows and, in rare cases, in piglets down to three weeks of age.

The economic effects of swine dysentery on a pig farm are devastating. The widely held view is that it is not a disease that can be lived with – it should be eradicated either by total herd depopulation, cleaning, disinfection and restocking with pigs declared free of the disease, by one of the many complex medication and cleaning eradication programmes, or, probably most attractive, by a combined approach (in other words, partial depopulation plus medication).

Treatment
If it is decided that diseased animals will be treated rather than destroyed, medication via feed or water with appropriate antimicrobials (such as the pleuromulins tiamulin or valnemulin) or lincomycin may be appropriate.

Prevention and Control
Once again, good hygiene practice to avoid the perpetual problem of faecal/oral recycling is an essential component of any control programme for swine dysentery.

Porcine Haemorrhagic Enteropathy (PHE)

This is a condition seen most frequently in growing pigs close to slaughter (in other words, five months of age) and in breeding stock up to one year of age, and is an acute form of ileitis, the disease caused by *Lawsonia intracellularis*

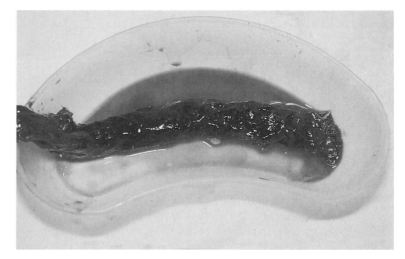

Fig. 54 A rope of clotted blood removed from the intestine of a grower pig that died of porcine haemorrhagic enteropathy (PHE).

(*see* page 62). It may even be some form of aller-gic reaction to the organism, but the result is sudden-onset massive damage to the lining of the intestine (mainly the lower small intestine and the large intestine), producing profuse haemorrhage in the gut lumen. This may pres-ent as a sudden-onset anaemia, the production of foul-smelling partially digested blood from the rectum (malaena; *see* Plate 4) or sudden death. At post-mortem examination, the par-tially clotted part-digested blood will form a 'rope' within the gut lumen, while the outside of the gut loops appear largely normal (*see* Fig. 54). It is unclear why some pigs react to *Lawso-nia* in this way, but it seems to be a condition associated with certain farms or herds, although on others it occurs as an outbreak, only to disappear as quickly as it came.

Treatment
When signs are noticed, the damage has already been done and the haemorrhage has occurred. Use of antibiotics such as lincomycin or tetracyclines may limit further damage but treatment is often unsuccessful. In an econom-ic environment, support therapies such as transfusion are unrealistic.

Prevention and Control
Prevention can be achieved by medicating feed with the above antibiotics over a risk period, although it remains to be seen what effect the *Lawsonia* vaccine will have on the incidence of this strange form of the disease.

Trichuris suis Infestation
This parasitic worm is an unusual cause of serious enteric disease in growing pigs that produces a scour indistinguishable from swine dysentery. It is seen most frequently, but not exclusively, in growing pigs kept in straw yards, and can also be involved in the complex syndrome of grower scours.

The life cycle of the parasite is direct – in other words, adult worms produce eggs (which are highly resistant to drying and disinfec-tion) that mature into infective larvae in the environment at a rate influenced by ambient temperature, and these then reinfect the pig and mature to adults in the gut. The life cycle can be quite short, allowing a rapid build-up of worms in the colon. Widespread scour with blood and mucus that is intractable to antibi-otic treatment or feed restriction is a telltale sign of *Trichuris* problems.

Treatment and Control
In an infected environment such as a straw yard, finishing pigs may require worming up to three times to prevent disease breakdown through *Trichuris* infection over a normal twelve-week cycle of growth. This often has implications with respect to withdrawal peri-ods of anthelmintics. To break the cycle of dis-ease, it is often necessary to depopulate a fin-ishing site of pigs, thoroughly wash and disinfect the area, then limewash all surfaces that have been in contact with the pigs. Only after the limewash has been left to cure for four days and the new incoming pigs have undergone a veterinary investigation or pre-cautionary worming to ensure they are free of worms should restocking take place. If worm-ing is not carried out until after the pigs have entered the area, there is still time for the pen or yard to be contaminated and hence the cycle of disease recommenced.

Volvulus/Torsion of Intestine
One of the most common causes of 'sudden' death in growing pigs is torsion of the intes-tine around its attachment to the dorsal body wall, known as the mesentery. The anatomy of this attachment in the pig is such that the gut is quite unstable, and if the intestine fills with gas this instability is increased and the whole intestinal mass can rotate 180 degrees or more, cutting off the blood supply. Death results within four hours and is characterized by pallor and abdominal distension. At post-mortem examination, the gut is distended and purple in colour, and contains liquid that is heavily tinged with blood (*see* Plate 5). Blood-stained fluid is also present in the free abdomen. The telltale sign of a torsion is that the caecum will point towards the head of the

pig rather than towards the pelvic inlet (*see* Fig. 55). Very occasionally, pigs will be seen alive. In such cases they will be depressed, lying on their sternum, often grinding their teeth, pale with distended abdomen and in respiratory distress. In such situations euthanasia is required.

The prelude to torsion (or twisting) is fermentation, and while certain dietary components have been implicated in this (for example, whey – particularly in winter – and high levels of soya), high feed levels and gorging are frequently associated with it. Diseases of the large intestine, such as grower scours, also have a strong association with fermentation and subsequent torsion.

Prevention and Control
Control of the condition lies in identifying and rectifying the trigger factors for fermentation. In some farms, however, occasional 'twisted guts' are the price paid for high feed intake and fast growth.

Gastric Ulceration
Part of the stomach of the pig is not glandular, but is lined with the same tissue as the oesophagus. This area is particularly prone to ulcerative damage, either at a microscopic level, leading to hyperkeratosis, or occasionally on a massive level, producing large ulcers that bleed into the stomach. The significance of low-grade damage is unclear, and a high proportion of pigs at slaughter show evidence of hyperkeratosis without apparently suffering ill effect. Here, we are more concerned with the dramatic haemorrhagic ulcer (*see* Plate 6).

Acid erosion is the cause of the haemorrhagic ulcer in pigs, unlike in human gastric ulcers, where *Helicobacter pylori* infection is implicated. Excess acid production and ulcers have been linked to specific dietary components (for example, wheat) and form (finely ground ingredients), dietary deficiency (vitamin E/selenium), and stress associated with environment, management and, in particular, concurrent disease (gastric ulceration is a common complication in pigs affected by *Actinobacillus*

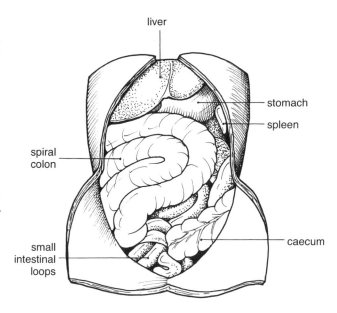

Note orientation of caecum and compare with Plate 5.
After Sisson and Grossman

Fig. 55 Topographic layout of abdomen of pig.

pleuropneumonia). Clinical signs range from sudden death, with the stomach full of clotted blood, to pallor and poor growth associated with tarry, foul-smelling faeces (malaena) as seen in PHE. The condition does occur in sows, which may show evidence of abdominal pain (hunched lying position, teeth-grinding).

Treatment
If the pig is alive when the condition is recognized, it should be hospitalized and given a high-fibre diet and reduced levels of hard feed. Secondary antibiotic cover is sensible, but it is better to avoid the use of non-steroidal anti-inflammatory analgesics (for example, ketoprofen) as these can exacerbate ulceration.

Prevention and Control
Control of a herd problem rests in identifying and correcting the primary causes.

Rectal Prolapse
Prolapse of the rectum is a common finding in both growing and adult pigs, and results from

inflammation of the terminal rectum or excessive straining. Thus, any lower bowel disease (for example, colitis, salmonellosis and swine dysentery) can be linked to prolapsing, as can constipation and the farrowing process in sows. The use of certain medicines (particularly tylosin and lincomycin) at high levels can also be associated with prolapse of the rectum. Probably the most common cause of prolapse in growing pigs is the pressure they exert on one another when huddling together in cold and draughty conditions. A pig that coughs when another is lying on its abdomen cannot release the abdominal pressure that occurs and the prolapse will 'pop out'. Spring and autumn therefore show a higher incidence of rectal prolapse in growers. Spontaneous prolapse also occurs in healthy, fast-growing weaners.

If the prolapse becomes damaged, the intestinal loops can themselves prolapse, in which case rapid death occurs. More commonly, the prolapse will be chewed off by pen-mates if it is not spotted in time; if this happens, a rectal stricture is a likely sequel (*see* below). The only sign of a chewed prolapse may be blood in the pen.

Treatment
If the prolapse is spotted early and the pig kept isolated it may be possible to replace the rectum with digital pressure. If the prolapse is severely enlarged (particularly common in sows) it can be shrunk by coating it with salt or sugar; this will allow it to be replaced more easily. If, however, it is damaged or cannot be replaced, amputation is indicated using the method illustrated in Fig. 57.

Prevention
Prevention of a rectal prolapse rests with identifying and correcting the underlying causes.

Rectal Stricture
Complete blockage of the rectum 2–3cm (1in) inside the anus is the result of scarring that occurs as a damaged or chewed prolapse heals,

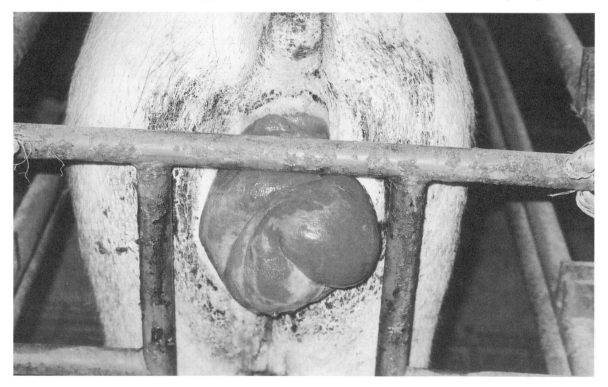

Fig. 56 Rectal prolapse in the farrowed sow.

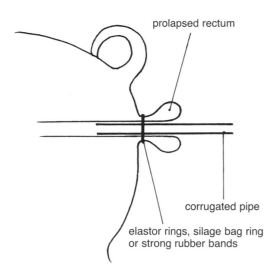

1. The corrugated pipe (e.g. 1in electricians conduit for growing pig) is inserted into the rectum through the damaged prolapse. Lubricate with obstetrical lubricant.
2. Place two rubber bands close to the perineum 'inside' the prolapse. The corrugation will help hold the pipe in place.
3. Within 5–7 days, the prolapse will have dried up and dropped off due to ischaemia and the pipe and bands will fall out.
4. Feeding castor oil during this time will assist voiding of faeces.

Fig. 57 Amputation of rectal prolapse.

whereby the ring of fibrous tissue slowly closes to obstruct the gut. Interruption to the blood supply of the rectum (associated with *Salmonella* and *Haemophilus parasuis* infection) can have a similar effect. Not all prolapses lead to stricture and not all strictures are seen as prolapses. Signs are progressive abdominal distension, loss of condition, hairy appearance and a gradually developing icterus (jaundice) as bile pigments are recycled from the gut (*see* Fig. 58).

Treatment
If spotted early, it is possible to expand the stricture digitally and hence allow the voiding of faeces in the short term, so that the growing pig can reach a slaughter weight. In most cases, however, the stricture is too advanced when seen and humane destruction is the only course of action available.

Intestinal Obstruction and Constipation
Obstruction of the gut can occur as an acute problem in the small intestine, and is caused by the presence of foreign bodies (such as stones) and dough balls, by very poor hygiene conditions and by massive *Ascaris suum* worm infestation (*see* Fig. 59). If seen alive,

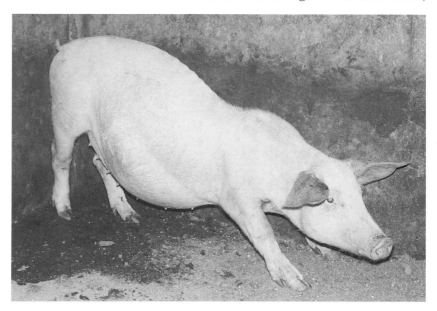

Fig. 58 Rectal stricture, producing faecal retention, abdominal swelling and loss of condition.

the pig will be depressed and is likely to be vomiting. Death is often the first sign in the commercial situation. Older growing pigs and sows outdoors are the most susceptible.

Constipation represents lower gut obstruction and is most frequently seen in sows around farrowing time. It may be a complaint of farrowing fever (*see* Chapter 4).

Treatment and Prevention
Acute obstruction tends to occur as a one off, except where *Ascaris suum* is involved, and here prevention lies in a combination of hygiene and worming programmes tailored to suit the circumstances. Liquid paraffin drenches can also be used to free a blockage (up to 4 litres/7 pints over forty-eight hours), while obstruction in sows prior to farrowing can be avoided by feeding bran mashes (*see* page 43).

Gastric Dilatation and Torsion

Uncontrolled expansion of the stomach with gas and its subsequent twisting is generally restricted to sows in confinement conditions such as stalls during pregnancy. It occurs rapidly and the sow is normally found dead with a massively distended anterior abdomen. There is a particular risk in sows fed small quantities of compound feed once per day. The condition appears to be linked with very rapid feed intake, possibly combined with the swallowing of large amounts of air, plus fermentation. In a dry sow stall or tether house in which the sows are fed manually, the greatest risk seems to be in those fed last.

Treatment
If the pig is still alive when the condition is noticed, exercise may help reduce the dilatation. However, if torsion (with or without the spleen) is involved, death will occur rapidly.

Prevention
Prevention can be achieved by increasing the volume of the diet (by using a low-specification high-fibre diet), feeding bulk forage (straw, sugar beet and so on) and feeding twice daily, and by installing automatic feeders that allow

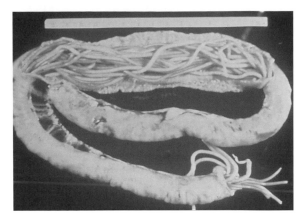

Fig. 59 Small-intestinal blockage due to Ascaris suum *worm infestation.*

simultaneous feeding. This condition is rarely seen in loose housing conditions in which straw bedding is used.

Other Conditions

The possibility of OIE (Office International des Épizooties) listed notifiable diseases (*see* Chapter 13) should not be ignored when making a diagnosis. With respect to enteric disease, classical swine fever (hog cholera) and African swine fever should be remembered in particular. Indistinguishable clinically, these two separate viral diseases cause widespread illness, with high temperatures in all age groups, nervous and respiratory signs, and vomiting, diarrhoea (with or without blood) and constipation. Haemorrhagic septicaemia is evident on post-mortem examination. Suspicion of either disease requires immediate notification to the appropriate authorities and, in most western pig industries, a slaughter policy is followed.

Diseases and abnormalities of the gastrointestinal system form a very large proportion of problems seen in the pig. Whilst many of these diseases are specific to pigs of certain ages, it would be a great error to make a diagnosis on age alone. Diarrhoea may be one of the most common clinical signs seen in a pig, but this chapter has highlighted other features of enteric disease.

CHAPTER SEVEN

Respiratory Disease

Diseases affecting the respiratory system of the pig constitute some of the most economically important ailments in commercial pig production worldwide. Although they are mostly diseases of the growing pig, they can affect a wide range of individuals. The principal signs that are seen with respiratory ailments are sneezing, coughing and difficulty in breathing (dyspnoea) in variable combinations, often associated with the more general signs of lethargy, inappetance and condition loss. An outline of the structure of the pig respiratory system is shown in Figure 60.

UPPER RESPIRATORY TRACT DISEASE

The upper respiratory tract consists of the nasal chambers, sinuses and nasopharynx. Damage and inflammation in this area produces a rhinitis. The nasal chambers of the pig contain scrolls of bone covered in mucous membrane called concha, which act to filter and humidify the air on its way to the lungs. Irritation of this area leads to sneezing and can result in damage that may compromise

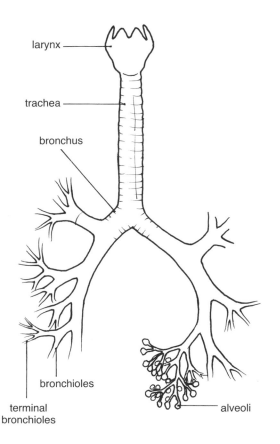

Fig. 60 Schematic structure of lower respiratory tract.

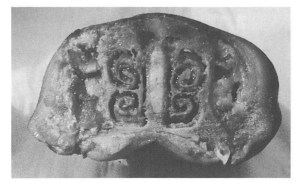

Fig. 61 The normal structure of the nasal chambers of a pig.

the filtration system and lead to secondary lung disease (pneumonia). There are a number of causes of rhinitis and, while most occur in the young pig, they can leave a legacy of damage into the growing phase.

Inclusion Body Rhinitis (IBR)

Also called porcine cytomegalovirus, IBR is caused by a ubiquitous virus (in other words, one that can infect the piglet prior to birth by transplacental spread). Most herds are thought to carry the virus and specific disease is rarely diagnosed. In a naive herd or litter, sneezing may occur within two weeks of birth and reduction in weaning weights will be seen. Severely affected pigs may die or be crushed by the sow. Secondary bacteria such as *Streptococcus suis* can infect the nose and produce a purulent discharge.

Treatment and Prevention
In most cases infection is asymptomatic, so no specific treatment is required. All in/all out farrowing practices and good hygiene may reduce the incidence of disease where it is seen.

Young Piglet Rhinitis

A common occurrence in commercial pig herds is sneezing (with or without coughing) in pigs aged fourteen days or more, which may lead on to more serious respiratory disease post-weaning (*see* porcine respiratory disease complex on page 83). Young piglet rhinitis may be associated with IBR infection but most commonly seems to be of bacterial origin, particularly those bacteria to which colostral immunity is not protective over a prolonged period – for example, *Haemophilus parasuis* and *Streptococcus suis*. Where pigs are reared in poor atmospheres (dusty and/or with high ammonia levels) the rhinitis may persist beyond weaning, but it does not usually produce lasting visible damage (in other words, the nasal conchae heal).

Treatment
Where the rhinitis is linked to bacteria such as *Haemophilus parasuis* and *Streptococcus*

suis, strategic medication of piglets by injection with long-acting antibiotics (for example, amoxycillin) at ten and twenty days of age is highly effective as long-term control.

Prevention and Control
Ensuring that piglets of varying ages are not mixed in the same air space through the adoption of an all in/all out system will reduce herd incidence of the disease.

Progressive Atrophic Rhinitis (PAR)

This is a specific infectious disease producing severe and permanent damage to the nasal conchae, such that, as the pig grows, the snout will distort upwards or sideways (*see* Fig. 62). The cause of PAR is infection early in life with *Pasteurella multocida* type D (rarely type A), resulting in a primary rhinitis. Sneezing and nasal discharges are seen in the suckling pig, but in severe cases nose bleeds (epitaxis) and ulceration of the gums and tooth roots can occur, limiting suckling. The nasal conchae will be irreparably damaged at variable rates, producing mild or severe loss of the filtering mechanism (*see* Fig. 63).

In extreme cases, where snout distortion has occurred, growth will be severely stunted – in an affected herd efficiency of growth can be depressed by more than 25 per cent. Deaths due to secondary pneumonia will also occur.

Treatment
In early cases of PAR, strategic medication given by injection at three, ten and seventeen days of age may limit the severity of the disease. Tetracyclines, penicillin and potentiated sulphonamides have all proved effective to a greater or lesser extent. However, as a major economic disease of commercial pigs, prevention of PAR is paramount.

Prevention and Control
Biosecurity measures should be designed to keep PAR out of a herd. Spread is solely pig to pig, and so liaison, coupled with quarantine, is needed to ensure incoming pigs are free. Seed-stock farms should be monitored for disease,

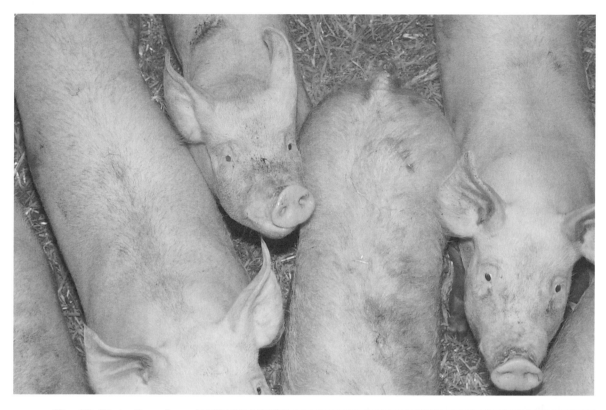

ABOVE: *Fig. 62 Distortion of the snout due to progressive atrophic rhinitis (PAR).*

Fig. 63 Total loss of the turbinate scrolls, and hence the nasal filter mechanism, through progressive atrophic rhinitis.

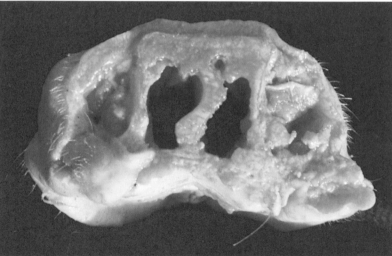

either by a snout scoring system in pigs at slaughter or by routine nasal swabbing of young growing pigs.

Where disease is known in an established herd, immunization of the breeding animals is required; a highly efficacious vaccine is available for this purpose. A primary course of two doses would normally be given prior to breeding, and then single booster doses prior to every subsequent farrowing. By controlling the primary agent of the disease (*Pastuerella multocida*), the co-infections (such as *Bordetella bronchiseptica*) that add to the damage are rendered impotent.

LOWER RESPIRATORY TRACT AILMENTS

The lower respiratory tract consists of the bronchi, bronchioles and the lung tissue, where exchange of oxygen and carbon dioxide between the bloodstream and air occur (*see* Fig. 60). In very general terms, insult to the airways produces irritation and coughing, whereas damage to the lung tissue (so called interstitial pneumonia) produces dyspnoea (*see* Figs 64 and 65). However, in practice, these differences are rarely discernible, with most specific and complex diseases producing both signs.

Enzootic (Mycoplasma) Pneumonia (EP)

Pneumonia caused by *Mycoplasma hyopneumoniae* infection, known as EP, is one of the most common types of porcine respiratory disease throughout the world. Primary infection occurs in the young pig, but clinical disease is most commonly seen between eight and twenty weeks of age as a low-grade cough and

slowed growth. In an uncomplicated form, the disease is mild and easily treated with antibiotics (tetracyclines are particularly effective). However, while *M. hyopneumoniae* principally causes interstitial pneumonia, infection does open the way for secondary bacterial disease, which produces bronchitis and a cough. With severe secondary infection, high temperature, severe depression and death can result. *Mycoplasma* infection is also a major component of the porcine respiratory disease complex (*see* page 83).

Mycoplasma hyopneumoniae is highly infectious and contagious, spreading from pig to pig by aerial transmission. It has been shown to spread 3–4km (2–2½ miles) on the wind and, hence, in areas of high pig density, infection and disease are ubiquitous.

Diagnosis
While the clinical presentation and herd background can give a presumptive diagnosis, *M. hyopneumoniae* infection can only be reliably confirmed at post-mortem examination. Figure 66 shows *M. hyopneumoniae*-damaged lungs at slaughter, when the presence of the bacterium can be demonstrated by PCR (polymerase chain reaction) testing. (An ELISA test is available on blood samples but currently is not specific enough to be definitive –

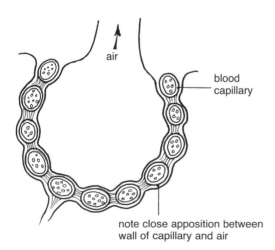

Fig. 64 Normal alveolus.

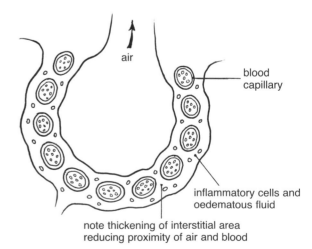

Fig. 65 Effect of interstitial pneumonia on alveolar structure and function.

Fig. 66 Apical lobe consolidation typical of Mycoplasma hyopneumoniae *infection.*

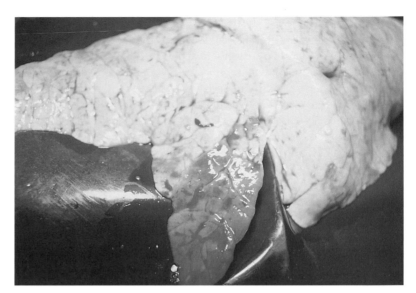

BELOW: *Fig. 67 Scoring system for enzootic pneumonia.*

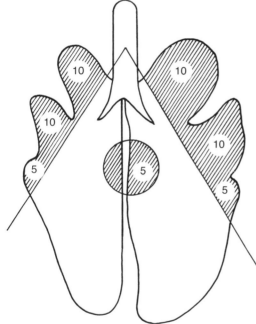

Each lobe that is shaded is given a score up to the maximum shown based on the proportion of tissue in the area that is affected – giving a maximum total of 55. (The unshaded area is not scored as it is rarely affected with enzootic pneumonia.) After Goodwin

lung damage can be assessed visually and a score out of 55 given for each animal (*see* Fig. 67) so that a herd score can be calculated. By looking at groups of fifty pigs, some idea can be gained of the impact of the disease on the herd. As a rule of thumb:

1. An average score of 4 or less suggests mild disease and is unlikely to justify herd intervention.
2. A score between 4 and 8 is significant and would justify intervention.
3. A score above 8 represents serious disease, in which mortality will be elevated and major intervention in terms of prophylactics and environmental adjustment are vital, both on an economic and welfare basis (5.5 points of damage equates to approximately 40g/1½oz per day lost growth in pigs weighing 30–100kg/65–220lb).

Treatment and Prevention

Mycoplasmas are very sensitive to appropriate antimicrobial agents (tylosin and tetracyclines) and long-term in-feed medication can be administered to suppress activity. Use of such antibiotics through water supplies, strategically targeted to precede clinical disease, can also be highly effective. However, the long-term use of

in other words, false positive results occur. This test is mainly used as a herd monitoring tool where slaughter animals are not available.) For monitoring purposes, the level of antibiotics is generally regarded as unacceptable and so other methods of control tend to be used instead. Of particular relevance here is the use of vaccination. *Mycoplasma* vaccines used on a herd basis are highly effective at inducing cell-medicated immunity, and herds that have used vaccines consistently for twelve months or more are normally found to have enzootic pneumonia scores of 2 or less (using 55 as the maximum, as above). A number of products are available, given as either one- or two-dose programmes, generally in the first three weeks of life. In particular, they are highly cost-effective in herds where enzootic pneumonia scores exceed 4. Combination vaccines containing *Mycoplasma* immunization are also available.

Alternatives to vaccination include the administration of high-dose antibiotics in the post-weaning phase (lincomycin and tilmicosin have both been used). Although this method is highly effective at 'clearing out' infection in the treated pigs, no lasting immunity occurs and so the pigs are vulnerable to reinfection. Such an approach is thus only applicable if the disease is to be eliminated from a herd or if the treated pigs are subsequently housed in isolation where reinfection is unlikely to occur. The other most important aspect of EP prevention is attention to environmental conditions (*see* page 84).

Actinobacillus pleuropneumoniae (APP)

This is one of the most severe pneumonias affecting the individual pig and, on a herd basis, can be devastating. In primary breakdown situations the disease can affect all ages, from adults right down to three-week-old pigs, but it is typically a disease of pigs aged ten to twenty weeks. Maternal, colostral protection will last up to nine weeks, thus leaving the growing pig vulnerable after this time.

At least twelve distinct serotypes of APP are recognized worldwide, although not all are present in every pig-keeping area. Each serotype is distinct and there is little cross-immunity between them. Moreover, each can be divided into a wide range of sub-types (biotypes), which can range from severely pathogenic to non-pathogenic.

The clinical picture is of a severe, rapidly progressing respiratory disease, with depression, inappetance, pyrexia (rectal temperatures above 42°C/107°F can occur), coughing and dyspnoea all evident. Death can occur so rapidly that well-conditioned pigs are found dead, often with bloody froth emanating from the nostrils. There will be purple discoloration of the extremities (ears, perineum and snout). At post-mortem examination, a severe necrotizing pleurisy and pneumonia is evident, with haemorrhage (infarction) within the lung tissue (*see* Plate 8). Occasionally, only one lung is affected. Death is a result of the combined effect of loss of lung tissue and toxaemia. Laboratory tests will isolate APP from untreated cases.

Treatment

As with many diseases, early recognition and prompt intervention are essential if a pig affected by APP is to be cured. Specific antibiotics (particularly ceftiofur) are highly effective and can give a remarkably rapid response. In addition, the use of non-steroidal anti-inflammatory agents such as ketoprofen and meloxicam can be valuable adjuncts to treatment by reducing pyrexia and reversing the effects of toxaemia. In an outbreak, prophylactic medication is needed and often must be given parentally, as the pigs may not take sufficient water to achieve satisfactory dosage via that route.

Long-Term Control

In an established herd, control must depend on breaking the cycle of infection between batches. This is discussed on page 84. As with *Mycoplasma* infection, treatment of young pigs with tilmicosin in feed can eliminate the organism but leaves the animal vulnerable to reinfection and, thus, is effective only if they remain in isolation.

Vaccination can be highly effective at reducing disease in a herd but, owing to the

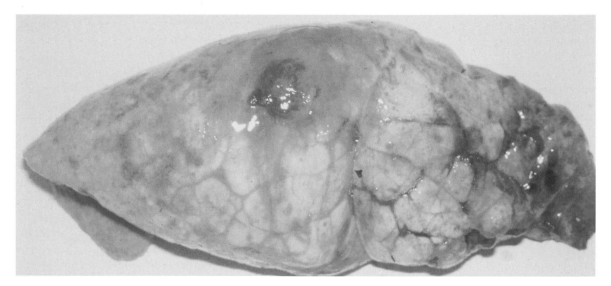

Fig. 68 Chronic Actinobacillus pleuropneumoniae *'core' lesions in the diaphragmatic lobe.*

variability of serotypes, it is necessary to match it with field strain. Multi-serotype vaccines do exist, although there are question marks over their efficacy. It is also possible – local regulations permitting – to produce an autogenous vaccine for a herd. Here, the actual causative isolate is used to manufacture a vaccine specifically for that herd's use. Such vaccines are normally given at around five and eight weeks of age. In most farm situations, single serotypes are involved but it is possible for more than one serotype to occur in any one population and, as such, autogenous vaccines need to take this into account.

Even in a vaccinated herd, lesions of APP may be evident at slaughter, usually as chronic abscesses or fibroid necrotic areas with overlying pleurisy (so-called 'core' lesions; *see* Fig. 68). It is not known whether the presence of such lesions will have had a significant economic effect on the pig. (Such lesions are grossly indistinguishable from those caused by *Actinobacillus suis* and can be differentiated only by laboratory testing.)

Monitoring
APP is a very widespread organism. Reports in the USA indicate that 80 per cent of herds are infected but only 20 per cent are affected – in other words, non-pathogenic biotypes are widespread. It is possible to monitor herds serologically although, again, ELISA tests are not specific and false positive results are common. Most seedstock producers will monitor the lungs of slaughter pigs and seek freedom from clinical and pathological signs (as opposed to aetiological freedom). It is thus difficult to maintain freedom from APP if pigs are being introduced, and the disease can be potentially explosive, particularly in situations where there is mixed infection with PRRS and/or swine influenza.

Glasser's Disease and *Haemophilus parasuis*
Glasser's disease caused by specific strains of *Haemophilus parasuis* is a septicaemic disease, while other strains of infection are more specifically targeted at the lung and respiratory system (*see* Fig. 69). More than twenty strains have been typed and many more untypable ones exist, the majority of them non-pathogenic.

Clinically, *Haemophilus parasuis* can cause disease from ten days of age, usually presenting as a cough. It is most significant, however,

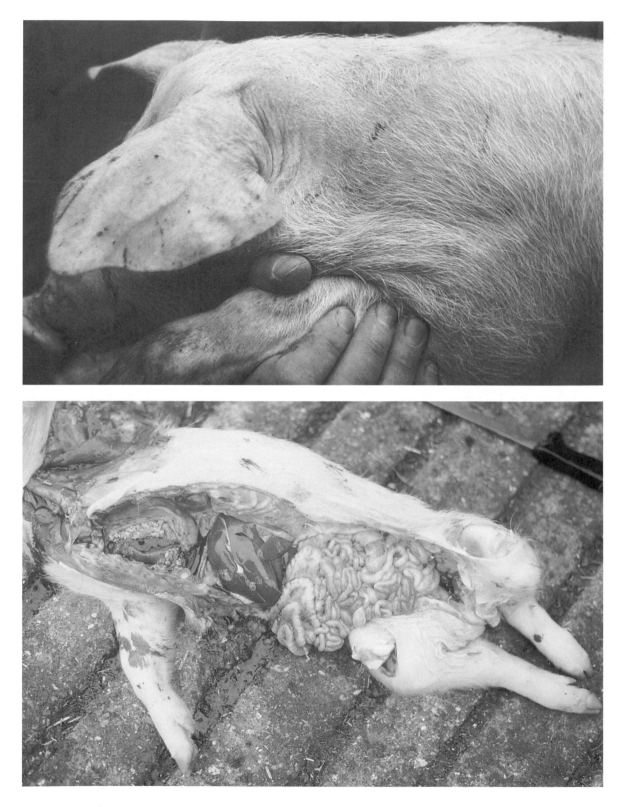

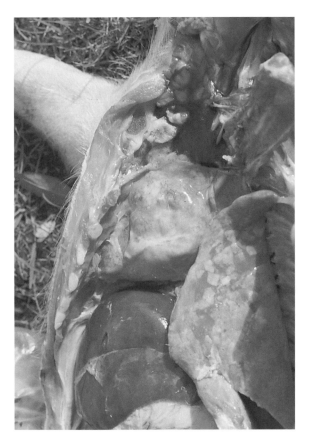

Fig. 71 Swollen pericardium typical of Glasser's disease.

OPPOSITE PAGE:
TOP: *Fig. 69 Acute clinical Glasser's disease, with hyperaemia of the ears and severe depression.*

BOTTOM: *Fig. 70 Acute Glasser's disease post-mortem, showing pericarditis, pleurisy and peritonitis.*

in the post-weaning period and, as an organism that is widespread in most pig populations, it is a common complication in other diseases, particularly PMWS, PRRS and EP. Signs of infection range from low-grade pneumonia (coughing and loss of condition) to sudden death with acute pleurisy. Pericarditis (in which inflammation of the sac surrounding the heart leads to constriction of the organ) is a common sequel and can account for sudden deaths in apparently recovered pigs.

Pericarditis lesions can also result from *Streptococcus suis* infection.

Treatment
Treatment of clinically affected pigs is extremely difficult and frequently unrewarding owing to the fact that, once evident, the damage is already done. The organism is particularly sensitive to penicillin and tetracycline but an accurate diagnosis is needed to target treatment.

The isolation of *H. parasuis* from a carcass is frequently unsuccessful owing to the fact that the lowering pH of the body kills off the organism. Likewise, any residual antibiotic treatment will render isolation unsuccessful. Sacrifice of an untreated affected pig and immediate processing in the laboratory are therefore needed to isolate *H. parasuis* reliably.

Prevention and Control
Prevention of the disease will depend on an accurate diagnosis and the age of the pig affected. Post-weaning medication via water or feed may be appropriate, and while vaccines are available caution is needed in their use. There is little cross-immunity between strains, and so a vaccine should be used only if the strains match. Moreover, colostral protection for *H. parasuis* is short-lived and disease may occur so early in life that it has not been possible to promote active immunity via a vaccine in time. As with all pig respiratory disease, pig flow, environment and management are critical to control.

VIRAL DISEASES

Swine Influenza Virus (SIV)
Swine influenza viruses are constantly evolving in the world pig population and there is an exchange of viruses between the pig, human and avian (particularly wildfowl) populations. Rural society in China is considered to provide a perfect medium for such an exchange and new strains of 'pig flu' are as likely as human strains. These pig flu strains may also cause disease in humans (in other words, they are

zoonotic). A common feature of influenza strains in the pig is that they produce a necrotizing bronchiolitis, the most significant sign of which is a severe cough.

In its classic form, swine influenza is an epizootic disease producing illness in pigs of all ages simultaneously, with pyrexia (40–42°C/ 104–107°F), lethargy and inappetance and a cacophonous cough widespread. Death is rare and the disease will normally disappear from a population within two to three weeks. Individual pigs recover without treatment in three to five days. The time taken to clear a herd will depend on the strain involved, the size and layout of the farm and weather conditions. Swine influenza appears to have a very strange ability to 'open the door' to other disease, particularly APP, and many outbreaks of the latter have occurred in herds previously clinically free following a brief influenza outbreak.

Severe herd outbreaks of swine influenza are typical of the strain H1N1195852, while milder, more vague disease can be seen in some circumstances. Often infection will effectively be asymptomatic in a *Mycoplasma*-infected herd, and it may only show up as a reproductive problem in sows that were infected at or soon after service. An increase in returns to service as a result of systemic infection – rather than specific reproductive infection – is common.

A chronic form of the disease is also seen in conjunction with PRRS infection of weaned pigs. As maternal immunity to both PRRS and SIV fades at four to six weeks of age, coughing and slowed growth will occur and secondary bacterial infection (by *Haemophilus parasuis* and pasteurellae) takes over. This particular manifestation (sometimes referred to as 'blue flu') is perpetuated where younger pigs are weaned in close aerial proximity to older affected animals – in other words, a vicious cycle of disease occurs. Breaking this cycle of reinfestation by altering pig flow is generally an effective long-term control strategy.

Prevention and Control
Swine influenza virus has been spread many kilometres on the wind, and as birds and man can also carry and spread the virus it is very difficult to exclude infection. However, in the absence of secondary disease, prolonged problems are rare. Biosecurity measures such as personnel down-time exclusions and bird-proofing the farm will be undermined by the presence of other pigs in the locality.

Vaccines against SIV are available in some countries but, due to the changing nature of the strains involved, they require regular updating in the same way as human flu vaccines. The cost benefit of vaccination would need to be carefully considered in the light of dubious or variable efficacy over the long term. Immunity to SIV in the individual is short-lived (a maximum of six to twelve months), which may have an influence on the decision to vaccinate.

Porcine Reproductive and Respiratory Syndrome (PRRS)
The reproductive effects of PRRS virus are dealt with in Chapter 1. Here, we are concerned with the respiratory effects of the virus, which now has a worldwide distribution following its initial outbreak in North America in the early 1980s.

Many herds are chronically infected with PRRS virus, but an immune stable breeding herd will convey immunity to the progeny that will last up to five or six weeks of age. Respiratory disease is typically seen on a herd basis from seven to ten weeks of age as a pneumonia. In an uncomplicated form, the disease is mild to indistinguishable and pigs will recover in less than a week with only a minor slowing in growth (*see* Fig. 72). However, when PRRS is present in conjunction with *Mycoplasma* and porcine circovirus, the effects are more dramatic and persistent as the secondary bacteria have added deleterious effects. Coughing, inappetance and loss of growth, combined with a steady mortality increase, are typical of the disease in weaners. And, as with all respiratory disease, infection is perpetuated where older affected pigs are in aerial contact with younger naive pigs.

The diagnosis of PRRS virus involvement in a respiratory outbreak can be achieved either

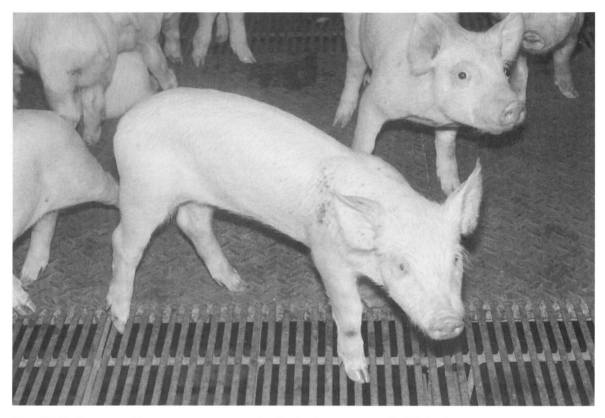

Fig. 72 Fading, coughing weaners as a result of mixed respiratory viral infection (swine influenza / PRRS) post-weaning.

by post-mortem examination with histopathology and immunocytochemistry tests or with PCR testing, or by blood sampling. In a PRRS-free herd, blood samples collected from survivors two weeks after the outbreak of clinical disease will confirm the involvement of the PRRS virus. In a known infected herd, viral activity must be demonstrated. In practice, this is best achieved by sampling a cross-section of the herd (for example, at three, six, nine, twelve and fifteen weeks of age) to show the point at which seroconversion occurs. Pigs born to immune sows are likely to have some residual immunity from colostrum at three weeks of age, although this will be lost by six weeks. Seroconversion by nine weeks of age is common and, if this corresponds to clinical disease at seven to eight weeks, a presumptive diagnosis can be made.

Treatment
Antibiotic medication will help control secondary bacterial infection and vaccination for *Mycoplasma* will reduce the impact of PRRS virus on the young pig. However, pig flow and environment are again critically important in breaking cycles of disease.

Prevention and Control
Vaccination of young pigs with live PRRS vaccines at around five weeks is highly effective at controlling primary infection, but on a herd basis it may be necessary to stabilize the breeding herd in addition to using respiratory vaccines. This will reduce the risk of viraemic pigs being born, which would otherwise act as a source of infection for others. (Other considerations with respect to herd control of the PRRS virus are detailed in Chapter 1.)

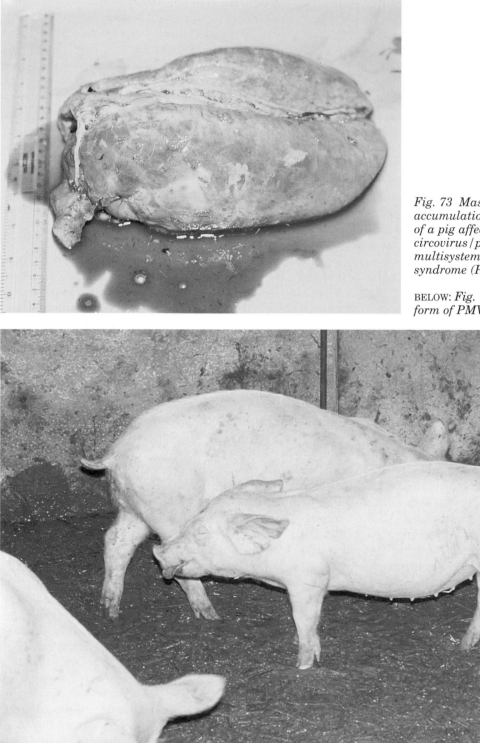

Fig. 73 Massive fluid accumulation in the lungs of a pig affected by acute circovirus/post-weaning multisystemic wasting syndrome (PMWS).

BELOW: *Fig. 74 The respiratory form of PMWS.*

Post-Weaning Multisystemic Wasting Syndrome (PMWS)

Enteric disease as a manifestation of PMWS is described in Chapter 6. However, in weaners PMWS can present as a respiratory disease and, in some herds, this can vary over time between the two major manifestations.

The true underlying causal aspect of PMWS remains unclear, but porcine circovirus type II is known to be involved in the pathology of the disease. This virus causes a severe interstitial pneumonia that interferes with gaseous exchange (*see* Fig. 65 on page 74). Severe dyspnoea results, and the effects of lung damage are exacerbated by a massive fluid outpouring into the lung tissue, producing oedema. Emaciated pigs aged six to twelve weeks with severe respiratory embarrassment are pathognomonic of PMWS, if such signs are combined with lymphadenopathy, particularly in the superficial inguinal region. That said, the disease should be confirmed histologically.

Prevention and Control

PMWS was first described in Canada in 1991 and has since spread around the world, such that few countries now remain free of the disease. Monitoring inevitably can only be done clinically – porcine circovirus type II is ubiquitous and has been so for at least thirty years. The control of PMWS is notoriously difficult and will certainly remain so until the true causative agent is identified. All that can be done at present is to minimize the effects of other disease, reduce stress and improve hygiene and comfort. Furthermore, breaking the cycle of reinfection between older and younger pigs is vital. Our understanding of this disease is continuing to evolve.

There is some evidence to suggest that herds affected for four to five years start to see a decline in incidence, and that progeny born to sows that themselves were reared as young pigs through PMWS disease (and survived and thrived) may be more resistant to the disease. This may explain the prolonged period that is apparently required for PMWS to burn itself out.

Porcine Respiratory Coronavirus (PRCV)

This is another very widespread agent within the pig population of the world, although some countries (for example, Ireland) have remained free of infection. In experimental animals, PRCV has produced severe and lethal pneumonia, but in the field disease is rarely identified.

The principal importance of this virus is in immunizing herds against the related transmissible gastroenteritis (TGE) virus, but its presence can interfere with international trade in pigs and pig products such as semen.

Aujeszky's Disease (AD, or Pseudorabies)

Aujeszky's disease (also known as 'mad itch') is caused by a herpes virus, which causes a wide range of clinical disease and tends to persist in a herd if not actively controlled. While reproductive and nervous signs predominate in older growing pigs and adults, rhinitis and pneumonia also occur, with sneezing and coughing the presenting signs. In countries where the disease is active and no specific control programme is in place, Aujeszky's should be considered as part of the respiratory complex in growing pigs. The disease is considered in both Chapters 1 and 8.

Prevention and Control

In an endemic situation, vaccination of both the breeding and feeding herd is necessary to effect control. Some regions and countries such as Great Britain and Denmark have eradicated this disease through national programmes. Others are working towards that goal by use of gene-deleted live vaccines and a combination of testing and removal.

Porcine Respiratory Disease Complex (PRDC)

There is a great danger when describing specific pig ailments that each disease is considered in isolation. However, in a farm situation, especially with mixed ages of pigs present, many diseases are of multiple aetiology and many of the agents described operate concurrently in the pig. This is particularly true of respiratory infections where a complex of PRRS virus, PMWS, *Mycoplasma*, Aujeszky's disease virus and secondary bacteria (including *Pasteurella*, *Haemophilus* and *Streptococcus*) combine to produce severe and often intractable problems known as porcine respiratory disease complex (PRDC). (The interaction between swine influenza and *Actinobacillus pleuropneumoniae* infection has already been highlighted on page 80.)

In order to understand what is going on in these complex situations, sophisticated diagnostic procedures are needed to clarify not only the agents involved but also the sequence of infection. On a herd basis, this will require detailed clinical appraisal, record analysis, serological profiles, post-mortem examination and abattoir assessment of slaughter pigs, along with histopathological techniques. Without such an approach, it is not possible to provide a definitive control strategy, although it is to this aim that we now turn.

CONTROL OF RESPIRATORY DISEASE

In terms of control of specific agents involved in respiratory disease outbreaks, an accurate diagnosis of agents involved is needed. Once this is known, specific control measures such as strategic medication and vaccination may be appropriate. However, some general control principles can be highlighted.

The recycling of disease within variably aged populations has been referred to many times in the preceding pages, and permanently occupied accommodation in which pigs of differing ages share air space will inevitably perpetuate respiratory disease (*see* Fig. 75). All accommodation should therefore be operated on an all in/all out basis, with age separation and routine cleaning between batches. Whether it is weekly production or batch production that is needed will depend upon the accommodation available. Taking this to the extreme, a multiple-site production – where pigs are weaned to dedicated remote sites each week – is a valuable tool for the larger herd, but in smaller herds the principle can be applied on a more modest basis, particularly outdoors (*see* Fig. 76).

Air quality is the other vital component of respiratory disease control. The individual pig has various protective mechanisms to prevent infection gaining access to its lungs. In addition to the nasal filtration mechanism discussed below, the main airways are lined with a 'mucociliary

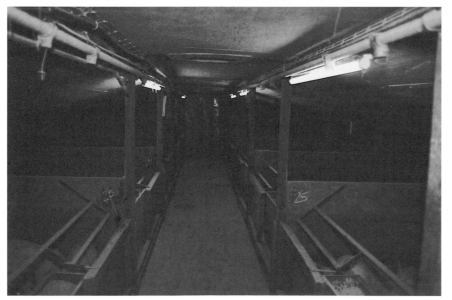

Fig. 75 Continually occupied buildings with a single air space provide perfect conditions for the persistence of respiratory disease.

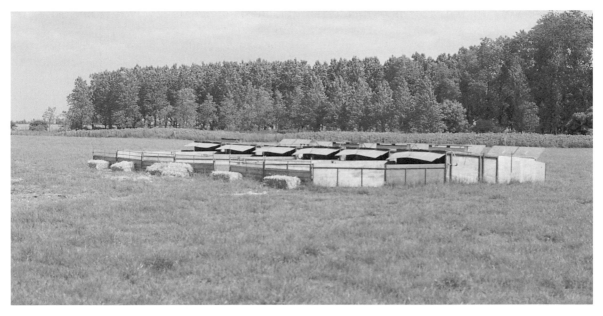

Fig. 76 Separation of weaner kennels into blocks to break the cycle of reinfection (the second block is in the top left-hand corner of the picture).

escalator'(*see* Fig. 77). Cilia on the surface of the cells lining the airways move the mucus upwards, such that it is then swallowed (this is phlegm). Anything that either overloads the mucous layer (such as heavy dust levels) or compromises the action of the cilia will

therefore reduce the clearance of mucus and potentially risk pneumonia. Aside from specific pathogens such as swine influenza virus, carbon dioxide will slow ciliary movement and high ammonia levels will paralyse cilia completely. In addition, high humidity and variable

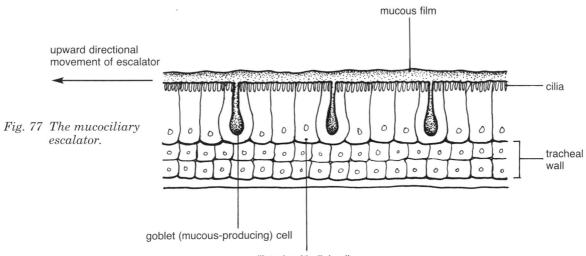

mucous film

upward directional movement of escalator

cilia

Fig. 77 The mucociliary escalator.

tracheal wall

goblet (mucous-producing) cell

ciliated epithelial cells

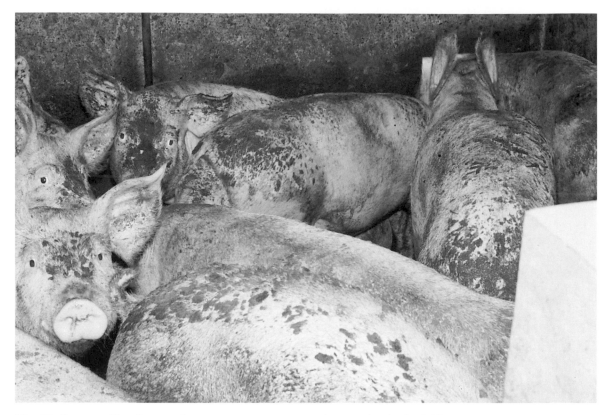

Fig. 78 Poor-quality dirty environments encourage respiratory (and other) disease.

temperatures upset the defence mechanism and precipitate disease, and stocking density is also critically important.

In a long-standing herd with chronic intractable disease, either total or partial depopulation is a useful technique to break the cycle of disease. In a partial depopulation all pigs are removed from the site from weaning onwards, and buildings are cleaned and refurbished; this therefore avoids a break in production from the breeding herd. Such an undertaking can coincide with treatment programmes in the sow to eliminate specific agents of *Mycoplasma* infection (*see* page 74).

OTHER CONDITIONS

It should not be forgotten that classical swine fever (hog cholera) and African swine fever cause respiratory disease *inter alia*, and so

these should always be considered where severe respiratory infection with mortality is seen. In such cases, other signs – such as reproductive failure and nervous disease – will normally be seen and the disease will affect all age groups. Similar comments would apply in instances of herd infection with Nipah virus.

Along with enteric diseases, ailments affecting the respiratory system of the pig are some of the most common problems seen in the field. The impact of respiratory disease can be measured in speed of growth, efficiency of feed utilization and mortality. The major infectious diseases that have been discussed in this chapter are responsible for enormous economic loss worldwide as well as representing a major welfare problem to the pig.

CHAPTER EIGHT

Nervous Diseases

The nervous system can be divided into the central and peripheral components. The central nervous system (CNS) comprises the brain and spinal cord, while the peripheral nervous system (PNS) consists of nerves running to all parts of the body, these carrying sensory stimulation and muscle control signals. Disease of the nervous system can affect either component and it is possible to locate where the nervous system is damaged by neurological examination. However, such a task is beyond the scope of this book and instead we will restrict ourselves to ailments that are easily recognized as affecting all or part of the nervous system. Locating lesions has limited practical application in the pig.

BACTERIAL DISEASES

Meningitis

The brain and spinal cord are protected within bony cavities (the skull and the spinal column, respectively), but separating the nervous tissue from the bone is a series of membranes

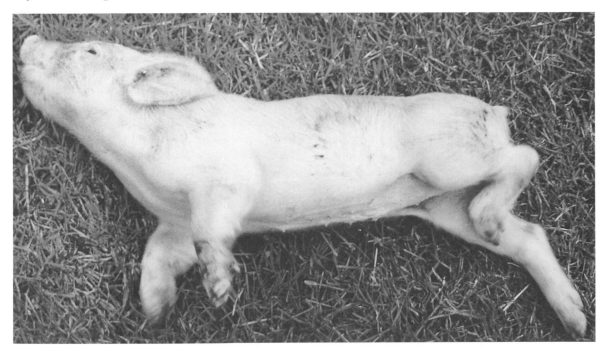

Fig. 79 Typical paddling convulsions in a pig affected with meningitis.

called the meninges. When these become inflamed in the condition known as meningitis (usually due to bacterial infection), pressure builds up on the nervous tissue and nervous signs ensue.

In the early stages of meningitis, pigs will be dull and depressed, reluctant to stand and have a raised rectal temperature. Occasionally, they may be seen pressing their head against a wall and they will be unsteady on their legs. As the disease progresses and in response to stimulation (handling, noise and so on), affected pigs will subside into paddling convulsions while lying on their side (*see* Fig. 79). Careful observation will reveal that the eyes, when open, will flick from side to side (this is called nystagmus). Death can ensue within a few hours and, indeed, some cases of meningitis may simply be found dead.

Infection in the brain results from blood-borne spread of bacteria, which can gain entry through any break in the skin or mucosa. Sporadic meningitis is particularly seen in the young piglet, where infection gains entry through the navel, tail-dock wound, clipped teeth or fight wounds, and is very much a feature of colostral insufficiency. Bacterial spread in the bloodstream (bacteriaemia) can lead to infection in other areas of the body – particularly the joints, causing joint ill, or arthritis (*see* Chapter 9). The bacteria involved are usually environmental contaminants such as staphylococci, *E. coli* and streptococci. However, epizootic forms of meningitis can occur in pig farms, particularly in weaner pigs four to ten weeks old and, rarely, in older growing pigs. The most common causes in these cases are *Streptococcus suis* type II and *Haemophilus parasuis*.

Streptococcus suis *Meningitis*

This is typically a post-weaning disease that is triggered by the stress of weaning and by mixing pigs of different ages. Overcrowding, poor ventilation and, in particular, high humidity all seem to exacerbate the disease. In an infected herd, the organism is picked up at or soon after birth, the reservoir being the nasal chambers and tonsils as well as the vagina of the sow. The organism colonizes the tonsil of the young pig and from there will spread via the bloodstream to the brain.

Onset of disease can be extremely rapid and sudden death may be seen. *Streptococcus suis* can readily be cultured from the meninges of an affected pig that has not been treated. Paddling convulsions are a classic feature, along with temperatures of 41°C (106°F) and above. The disease usually behaves in an all or nothing way – in contrast with most gut or respiratory tract diseases, there is no effect on the growth of unaffected meningitic pigs.

There are many sub-strains of *S. suis* type II, all with varying pathogenicity. Where particularly severe strains occur, control can be difficult – vaccines have not proved effective and strategic use of antibiotics such as amoxycillin or ceftiofur by injection at weaning may be needed to prevent clinical disease. Medication of weaned pigs via water or feed with penicillin-based antibiotics will often suffice in milder outbreaks. Recovered pigs may drop dead suddenly two or three weeks later, the result of seeding of infection on the heart valves and production of endocarditis (*see* Chapter 11).

It should be remembered that *S. suis* type II (along with other strains of *S. suis*) are zoonotic, so particular care should be taken when handling affected pigs and when attending farrowing in herds known to be infected. Infection for humans is normally by skin penetration through cuts and grazes – thorough hand washing with soap is essential following contact with potentially infected material.

Haemophilus parasuis *Meningitis*

Glasser's disease caused by *Haemophilus parasuis* infection was discussed in detail in Chapter 7. There are many strains of *H. parasuis* present within pig populations and, while the most common manifestations of disease are either respiratory or septicaemic, cases do occur where the infection targets the brain, producing meningitis (arthritis is also occasionally seen). The clinical presentation is identical to that described above, but diagnosis can be difficult as the organism is very fragile post-mortem – euthanasia of an affected untreated pig and immediate sampling of the meninges or cerebral spinal fluid is essential.

Treatment

Treatment of any form of meningitis is based upon killing the causative organism and providing support therapy. *Streptococcus suis* is generally very sensitive to antimicrobial treatment with penicillin-based medicines such as amoxycillin, but treatment must be rapid and involve a formulation that achieves high levels of antibiotic in the body immediately. Long-acting preparations often give disappointing results. While *Haemophilus parasuis* is also very sensitive to antibiotics, response to treatment of affected pigs is frequently disappointing, probably due to the fact that clinical signs are the result of toxin release rather than the effect of the bacterium itself; by the time signs are seen, the damage is done and killing off the organism will have no effect.

A common complication of meningitis in pigs is dehydration. Their inability to feed and drink soon leads to fluid shortage, especially in the young pig. This is often manifest in the form of 'salt poisoning' (water-deprivation neuropathy), which can easily be confused with meningitis clinically even though it is quite distinct from it. Thus, many pigs that die through meningitis infection actually subside into salt poisoning, which is the true cause of death. (Salt poisoning is discussed in more detail on page 95.)

To prevent such complications, it is necessary to provide active nursing to a meningitic pig. The animal should be removed from the pen – where it would be attacked by others – and placed in a bedded area to prevent injury. Often, response to treatment will be very rapid (within two to four hours) and, therefore, it may be reasonable simply to move the pig to the passageway, reintroducing it to the pen when it has recovered. It should be given fluids (water containing electrolytes), preferably by mouth on a little and often basis. Care must be taken to ensure that the pig is swallowing fluids and not inhaling them.

If the swallowing reflex is lost or if handling the pig in order to give it a drink stimulates excessive convulsions, fluids can be provided per rectum. Using soft silicone tubing, the tube is inserted with generous lubrication into the anus and, in a pig of 6–10kg (13–22lb), can be passed up to 10–15cm (4–6in) into the rectum. This must be done gently to avoid penetrating the rectum. Up to 50ml of warm fluids can then be 'injected' up the tube. This should be repeated every two hours until the pig is able to drink for itself.

Support treatment with corticosteroids or non-steroidal anti-inflammatory agents can also improve recovery rates. As a general rule, however, a failure to respond to treatment within forty-eight hours is likely to leave the pig permanently brain-damaged and so euthanasia is appropriate.

Bowel Oedema

Post-weaning *E. coli* diarrhoea is discussed extensively in Chapter 6. A specific manifestation of this disease is bowel oedema, which is associated with nervous signs.

Bowel oedema was an extremely common condition up until the 1970s, particularly in pigs that were weaned late (at five to six weeks). Since then, outbreaks have been unusual and sporadic, even though specific *E. coli* strains (for example, E68 II) have remained prevalent. Where the condition does occur, it is typically seen within two to three weeks of weaning and may or may not have been preceded by a bout of scouring in the group of pigs.

Onset of disease is sudden, and the pig may be found collapsed or dead. If alive, it will emit a classic high-pitched squeal – the result of fluid accumulation in the vocal cords – and will be totally uncoordinated if it tries to stand or walk. Swelling of the head is typical as a result of fluid accumulation (oedema) under the skin. At post-mortem examination, oedema is evident in the support structures of the intestine (the mesentery). Diagnosis is based upon clinical signs and post-mortem findings, and can be supported by histopathological examination of the brain and isolation of

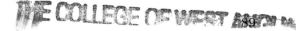

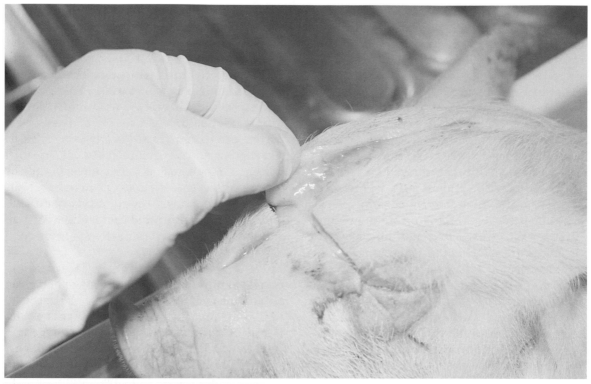

ABOVE: *Fig. 80 Subcutaneous oedema of the head, associated with bowel oedema.*

Fig. 81 Fluid accumulation in the mesentery of the large intestine, seen in cases of bowel oedema.

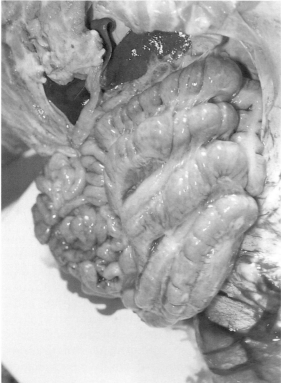

haemolytic *E. coli* strains (which contain the 'oedema' toxin) from the gut.

Treatment
Treatment of affected pigs is usually unsuccessful. As with *Haemophilus parasuis* meningitis (*see* above), killing the causative organism will have no effect as the damage will already have been done by the toxins present. Attempts to reduce the oedema by use of diuretics appear to be frustrated by difficulties in maintaining the correct fluid balance – salt poisoning is a high risk where such medicines are used.

Prevention and Control

Concentration on dietary management is required to prevent the condition. Engorgement with food post-weaning appears to be the major trigger factor and so attention to feeding little and often – to the point of severe restriction – may be needed, particularly in late-weaned pigs. Use of selected antimicrobial agents in water in anticipation of clinical disease and targeted injection with, for example, fluroquinalone antibiotics prior to expected disease (metaphylaxis) is highly effective. The inclusion of high levels of zinc (in the form of zinc oxide) in post-weaning diets will suppress *E. coli* growth, as will in-feed antibiotics but, due to the nature of *E. coli*, antibiotic resistance will soon occur. Inclusion of organic acids in weaning diets may also limit *E. coli* proliferation in the gut.

Middle Ear Disease

The balance mechanism for the body is contained within the inner part of the ear (*see* Fig. 82). Any disturbance to this mechanism will therefore affect balance and coordination. The most common abnormality is infection, initially of the middle ear, which exerts pressure on the balance mechanism. There are two distinct phases to the disease:

1. In the early stages of the first phase, damage is limited to the middle ear. The pig will frequently shake its head and, as it stops, the head will be left tilted to one side with the affected ear downwards. The head will then slowly return to normal. This phase is frequently ignored by stockmen as the pig appears to recover.
2. In the second phase, damage occurs to the inner ear and a permanent head tilt results. Head shaking may still be frequent, and the pig may be unsteady and tend to walk in a circle. In severe cases, the pig will have difficulty eating, drinking and competing with penmates, and loss of condition will occur.

There are a number of potential causes of middle ear disease. Infection with opportunist organisms can occur either from the external ear canal following penetration of the tympanic membrane (eardrum), or via the Eustachian tube from the oropharynx. The former is particularly associated with mange infestation in growing and young adult pigs, whereby rupture of the tympanic membrane is either a direct result of the mites or secondary to head shaking. Rough handling (lifting pigs by the ears) can also damage the tympanic membrane and allow penetrating infection.

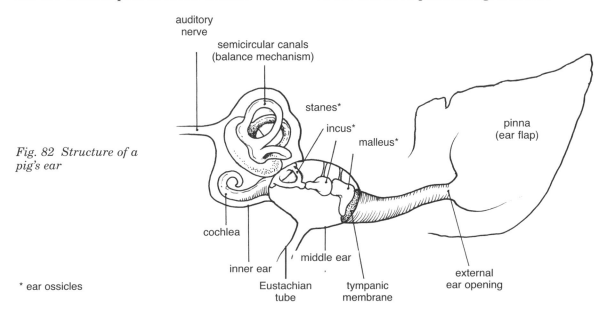

Fig. 82 Structure of a pig's ear

auditory nerve

semicircular canals (balance mechanism)

stanes*

incus*

malleus*

pinna (ear flap)

cochlea

inner ear

Eustachian tube

middle ear

tympanic membrane

external ear opening

* ear ossicles

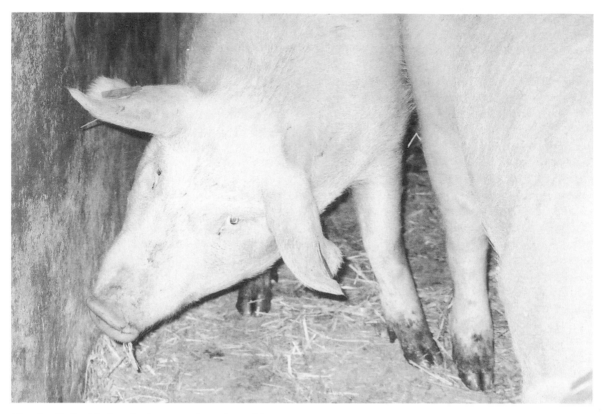

Fig. 83 Left-side head tilt in a gilt with middle/inner ear disease.

The oropharynx is normally colonized by a wide range of organisms, which potentially can spontaneously ascend the Eustachian tube, particularly in young growing pigs. However, inflammation of the oropharynx as part of any upper respiratory tract disease will predispose the animal to such ascending infection. This is particularly seen in association with swine influenza, where outbreaks of middle ear disease have occurred one to three weeks after an influenza outbreak in growing pigs.

Studies in the USA have consistently isolated *Mycoplasma hyorhinus* from cases of middle ear disease, but frequently streptococci and staphylococci are also found.

Treatment
Broad-spectrum antibiotics (synthetic penicillin or potentiated sulphonamides) administered in the early stages for a prolonged period

of five to seven days will bring about a complete cure. However, the more developed the case, the more difficult it is to effect successful treatment, and the pig may be left with a permanent head tilt. Provided it is steady on its legs, is clear of antibiotics, does not have a raised temperature and is of sufficient size, slaughter as a casualty animal is appropriate. Severe cases will almost certainly require euthanasia.

Spinal Abscessation
Abscesses in the spine are a common complication of tail-biting, which usually occurs in the thoracolumbar area. The effect of such biting is to exert pressure on the spinal cord such that paralysis distal to the abscess occurs. In practice, this means that the pig will go off its back legs and will be both faecally and urinary incontinent. Affected pigs

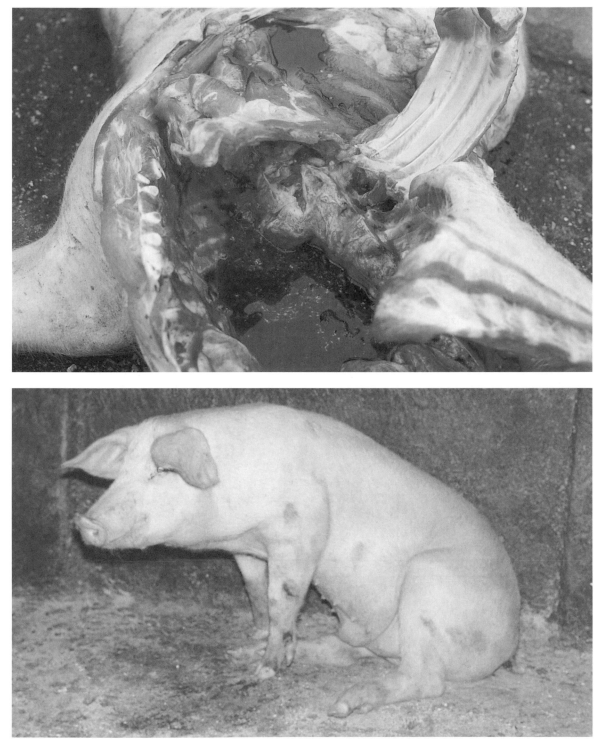

TOP: *Fig. 84 Abscessation near the spinal column secondary to tail-biting.*

ABOVE: *Fig. 85 Posterior paralysis typical of a spinal abscess.*

will often drag themselves around by their front legs and be able to feed and drink, and so can survive for an extremely long time. Clearly, euthanasia is appropriate at the earliest indication of loss of use of the hind legs.

Arcanobacterium pyogenes (formerly called *Actinomyces pyogenes*) is the most frequently isolated organism responsible for the development of abscesses. Contrary to popular belief, the infection does not ascend the spine directly but is spread in the lymphatic duct, which runs under the spinal column. (Tail-biting as a primary condition is dealt with in Chapter 10.)

Treatment

Treatment of tail-bitten pigs with broad-spectrum antibiotics will help prevent secondary infection such as spinal abscesses. However, once formed, these abscesses are practically untreatable; even if clinical recovery can be achieved, a residual lesion will remain that will require whole carcass condemnation at slaughter.

Tetanus

Clostridium tetani is a soil-borne bacterium that invades contaminated wounds. It then proliferates at that site, producing and releasing a powerful neurotoxin that causes excessive muscle contraction without subsequent relaxation. Tetanus can potentially affect pigs of all ages but is most frequently seen in the young pig outdoors on land that is known to be contaminated with *Clostridium tetani*. Other species in the proximity may also succumb.

Castration is probably the most likely precursor to disease, with soil contamination of the wound resulting in tetanus approximately three to four weeks later. The clinical signs are absolutely typical:

1. Lateral recumbency, with the legs held rigidly pointing backwards but no paddling motion.
2. The back will be arched and the head held back over the shoulders (opisthotonus).

3. The ears will be held pricked and the tips will be curled over.
4. The tail will be held straight out.

In extreme cases, it is possible to lift the pig by one leg so that the whole body is rigidly held out, stiff as a board.

Treatment and Prevention

Practical treatment of affected piglets is not viable and euthanasia is appropriate. In high-risk situations (for example, on known infected land) where invasive procedures are required – particularly castration – tetanus antitoxin should be administered at the time of invasion (2000IU per piglet).

VIRAL DISEASES

Aujeszky's Disease (AD, or Pseudorabies)

This herpes virus of pigs is described in Chapters 1 and 7. It is, however, a disease of complex pathogenesis and the signs will vary with the age of pig affected and the dose of infection acquired. Nervous signs are normally restricted to suckling and young growing pigs. The suckling pigs will show muscle trembling, depression, circling, lack of coordination and a typical dog-sitting position. Over a period of one to two days, this will progress to collapse and convulsions, followed by death. In weaners and young growers, the disease may have a slower progression and present more in the form of muscle spasm and incoordination of the hind legs, before leading to convulsion, coma and death. In all cases, temperatures will be raised to 40–41°C (104–106°F).

Prevention and Control

Control of Aujeszky's disease is based on whole farm, regional or national programmes involving vaccination, testing and removal or compulsory slaughter. Many pig-producing countries are now free of the disease and most countries of the EU are working towards a similar status.

Enteroviruses

Teschen and Talfan are caused by related – if not the same – enteroviruses and, while serological evidence of these viruses is widespread, disease is uncommon.

Teschen is a severe polioencephalomeningomyelitis, producing incoordination, irritability and stiffness of muscles in association with a raised temperature, subsiding into convulsions, paralysis and death over a period of three to four days. This form of the disease is not seen in western Europe but is widely reported in central and eastern parts. Talfan, meanwhile, occurs as a mild sporadic disease in young piglets, producing a slight fever followed by hind-limb ataxia and paralysis with dog-sitting, which is usually irreversible. Animals rarely die but euthanasia is appropriate.

Prevention and Control

Teschen used to be a notifiable disease under EU legislation and slaughter remains the likely method of control. Vaccination is practised using live attenuated vaccines in parts of eastern Europe.

There are no specific control measures for Talfan, but it should be noted that, while infection appears to be ubiquitous and, therefore, disease is only likely to be seen in young piglets with inadequate immunity, the modern practice of split-site production (where the breeding herd, nursery and finishing sections are physically separated) could allow the virus to 'burn out', leaving gaps in immunity. Likewise, inadequate integration and acclimatization of gilts coming onto a farm (particularly if they have been derived from split-site production systems) may also allow non-immune animals to enter the herd and naive progeny consequently to be produced.

Exotic Viruses

A range of other viruses exists that, when present in pig populations, can cause widespread disease in all age groups, these including nervous signs.

Classical Swine Fever and African Swine Fever

These used to be listed under the Organisation International des Épizooties (OIE) List A of exotic diseases, for which compulsory control measures exist (*see* Chapter 13).

Japanese B Encephalitis

A mosquito-borne viral disease of pigs (and other species, including man) restricted to South-East Asia and the Pacific Rim. It produces both reproductive and nervous disease.

Nipah Virus

This is a commensal virus of fruit bats in Asia that has crossed over to pigs to produce a severe and fatal nervous disease. A major outbreak in Malaysia in 1998/9 led to the slaughter of half the pigs in that country. The disease is particularly significant in that it can also pass to man – in the Malaysian outbreak, more than 100 in-contact pig workers died from Nipah virus infection.

POISONINGS

A wide range of potential poisons – including plants, heavy metals and miscellaneous chemicals – can cause a range of nervous diseases in pigs. It is beyond the scope of this book to detail all of them, but a summary is provided in Figure 86. However, the most common and economically important poisonings do require some explanation.

Salt Poisoning

More accurately, this condition is called water-deprivation neuropathy and arises as a consequence of dehydration. The affected pig appears particularly susceptible to suffering neurological damage, which is only rarely seen as an effect in other species. The pathogenesis of salt poisoning is a two-step process:

1. A reduction in body fluids leads to dehydration of the brain, with the result that salt concentration (sodium and chloride ions) increases. This has the direct effect of producing eosinophilic meningoencephalitis,

Poison	Potential sources	Effects
Arsenicals	Feed medication, insecticides, herbicides	Ataxia, 'goose-stepping', blindness, convulsions, death
Lead	Paint, car batteries	Blindness, constipation, blood poisoning
Mercury	Dressed grain, fungicides	Ataxia, blindness, paresis, coma (terminal)
Nitrofurans (e.g. furazolidone)	Medication	Ataxia, paresis (reversible)
Chlorinated hydrocarbons	Insecticides (e.g. lindane dieldrin)	Hyper-excitability, muscle spasms, tremors
Strychnine	Mole bait	Hyper-excitability, photophobia, tetanic spasms, rapid death
Amaranthus (pigweed)	Pasture/hedgerows	Weakness, trembling, knuckling, post-paresis, death in forty-eight hours
Deadly nightshade	Pasture/hedgerows	Pupil dilation, trembling, paddling convulsions, death

Fig. 86 Sources of selected poisons and their effects.

which is associated with neurological disorder. Depression, collapse and opisthotonus are the most common signs but, significantly, there is no elevation of body temperature.

2. More dramatic disease is seen following rehydration. The elevated salt concentration in the brain exerts an osmotic draw on fluids, which consequently flood into the brain to produce oedema (fluid swelling). This is accompanied by a dramatic onset of nervous disease, which is typified by affected pigs falling over backwards. They tend to stagger back, drop into a dog-sitting posture, throw their heads back over the shoulders (opisthotonus) and tumble backwards. They may then subside into convulsions, after which death will occur rapidly.

The initial concentration of salt in the brain can arise through several means:

1. Very high salt levels in the feed without providing adequate water. This is particularly a risk where waste/by-product feed is used and no supplementary water is supplied.

2. Interruption of water supply as a result of mechanical fault, freezing pipes or excess competition.
3. Inadequate water intake as a result of other disease (e.g. meningitis or lameness).
4. Excessive fluid loss due to diarrhoea.

The 'flooding' of the brain is the direct result of supplying water to pigs that have previously had restricted intake or have suffered salt concentration. The classic picture is of pigs whose water supply has been frozen over for a weekend, the situation being remedied only on the Monday when water is offered. In this case, a few pigs may be depressed initially but, as the majority start to drink, clinical signs develop within minutes.

Treatment
Treatment of salt poisoning relies on the ability to rehydrate the pig gradually. This can be done either by offering very small amounts of water orally over a prolonged period, providing snow for the pigs to eat or by injecting fluid into the peritoneum (50–100ml per 20kg/45lb, repeated

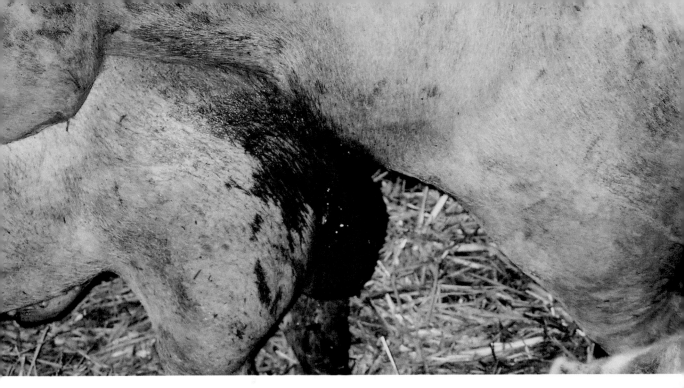

ABOVE: *Plate 1 Damage to the penis in the boar usually results in haemorrhage.*

RIGHT: *Plate 2* Clostridium perfringens *type C: acute haemorrhagic enteritis.*

BELOW: *Plate 3 Swine dysentery causing a haemorrhagic colitis.*

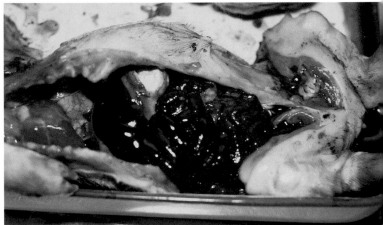

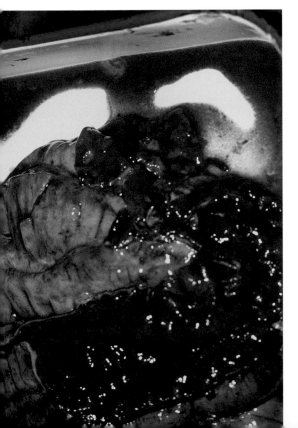

BELOW: *Plate 4 Digested blood produced from a pig with porcine haemorrhagic enteropathy (malaena). The colour of the blood is distinctive and is accompanied by an unmistakable smell.*

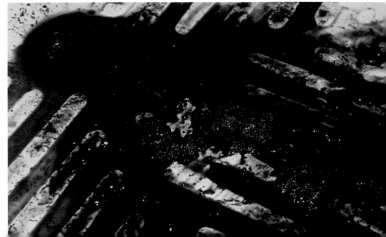

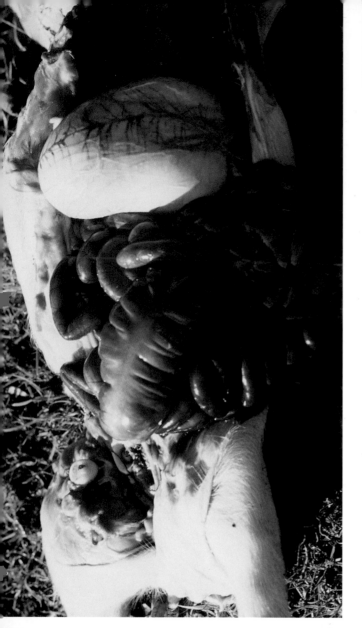

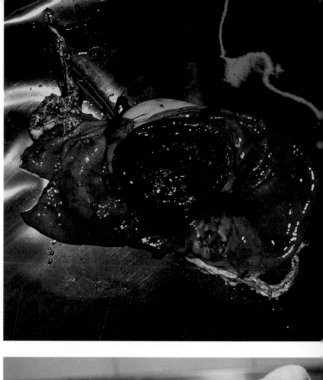

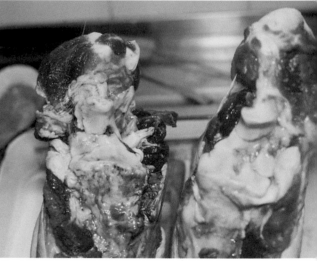

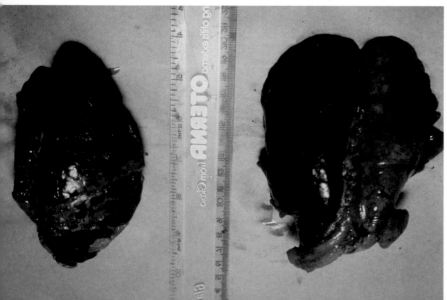

ABOVE LEFT: *Plate 5 Volvulus or twisted gut, producing gas-filled gangrenous gut loops (note the layout of the intestine compared to the 'normal' state depicted in Figure 55, page 67).*

TOP: *Plate 6 Gastric ulceration can be so severe as to cause death through haemorrhage.*

ABOVE: *Plate 7 Osteochondrosis of the joints, showing erosion and deformation of the cartilage.*

LEFT: *Plate 8 Acute* Actinobacillus pleuropneumoniae *infection producing haemor-rhage, infarction and pleurisy.*

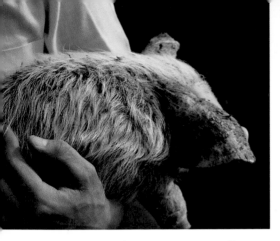

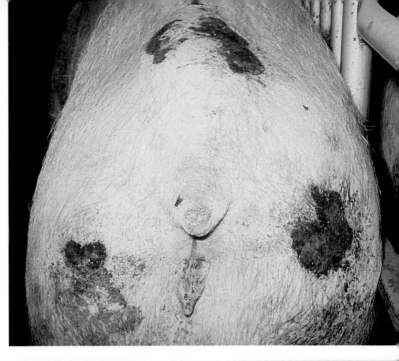

ABOVE: *Plate 9 Classic greasy pig disease in a weaner pig.*

RIGHT: *Plate 10 Ulcerative greasy pig disease.*

BELOW: *Plate 11 Chronic greasy pig disease in a grower pig.*

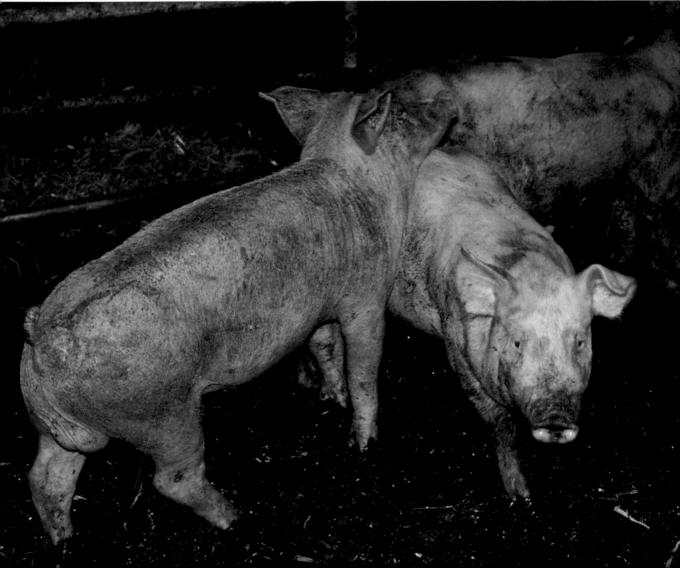

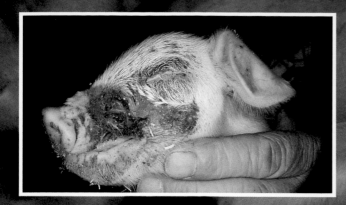

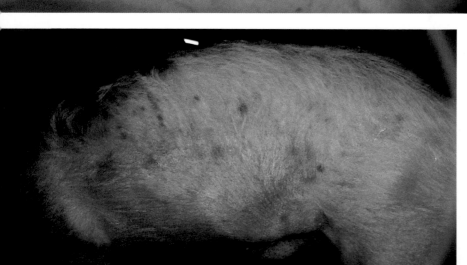

INSET: *Plate 12 Oral necrobacillosis resulting from a failure to clip teeth.*

ABOVE: *Plate 13 Acute erysipelas – note the diamond-shaped lesions on the back.*

LEFT: *Plate 14 Pig pox in a weaner pig.*

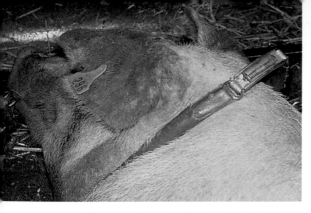

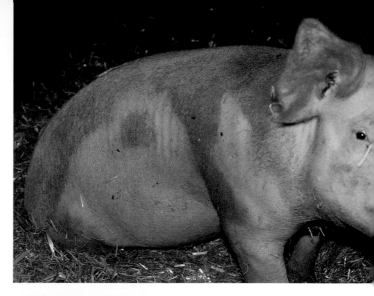

ABOVE: *Plate 15 Acute PRRS producing the eponymous 'blue ear'.*

RIGHT: *Plate 16 Skin discoloration is also seen with acute PRRS.*

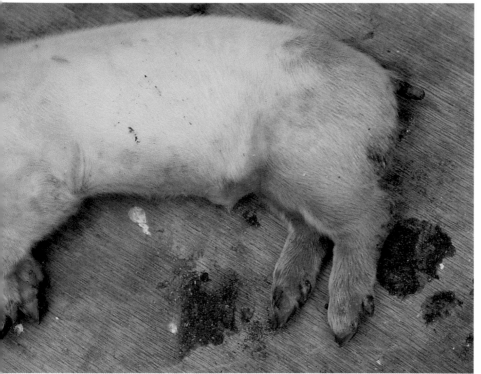

LEFT: *Plate 17 Bruising following iron injection in a young piglet.*

BELOW LEFT: *Plate 18 Acute porcine dermatitis nephropathy syndrome (PDNS) producing intradermal haemorrhages.*

BELOW: *Plate 19 Mange infestation.*

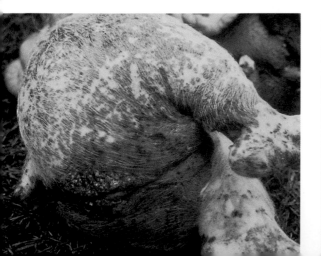

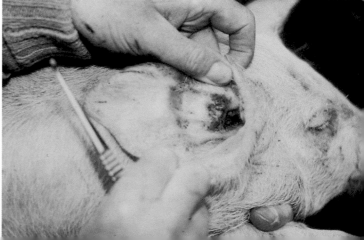

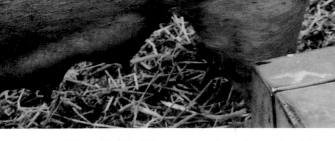

TOP: *Plate 20 Fly bites can produce dramatic skin lesions as well as spreading disease.*

ABOVE: *Plate 21* Trichophyton mentagrophytes *produces lesions that look more like dirty marks than the classic signs of ringworm (see Figure 114).*

RIGHT: *Plate 22 Pityriasis rosea in a weaner.*

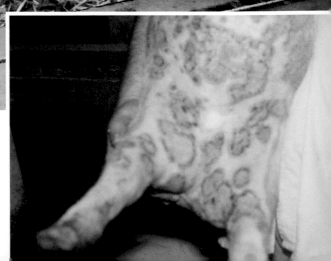

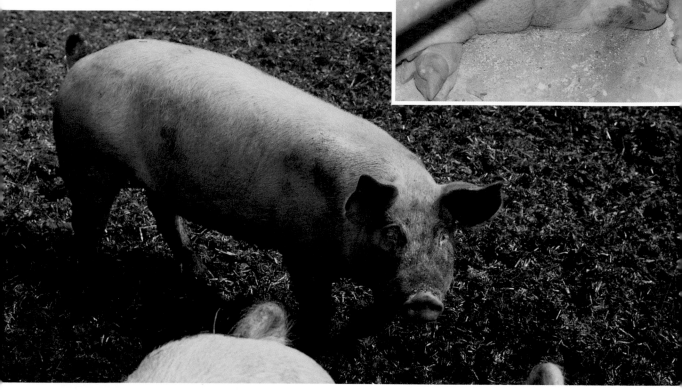

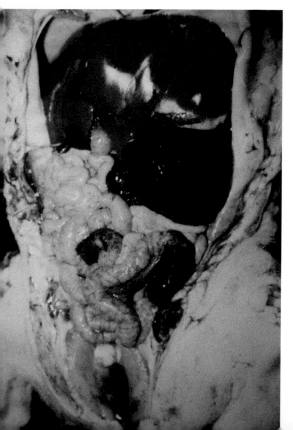

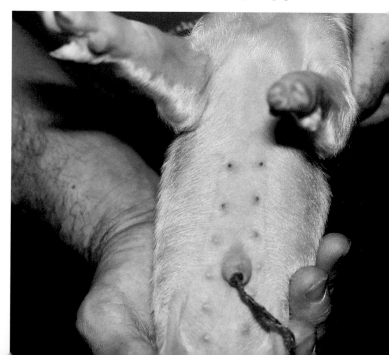

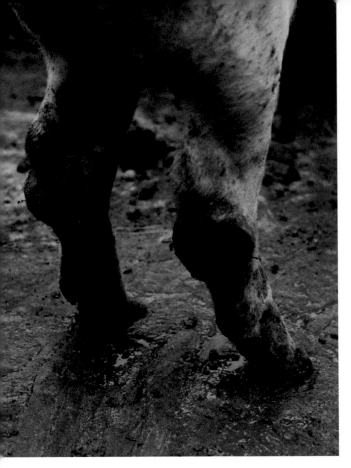

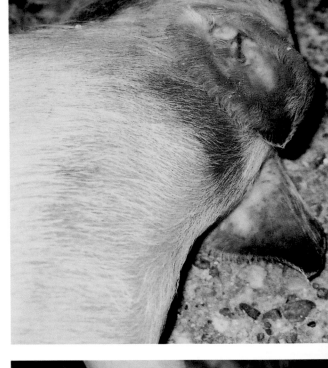

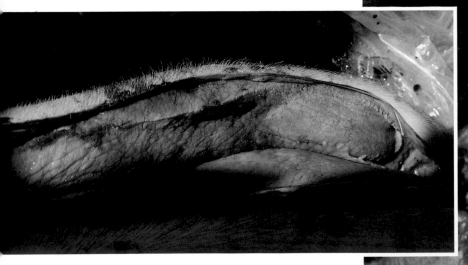

ABOVE: *Plate 27 Ulcerative bursitis in a grower pig.*

ABOVE RIGHT: *Plate 28 Acute septicaemia with hyperaemia of the extremities.*

ABOVE: *Plate 29 The semi-cooked appearance of muscle following death due to porcine stress syndrome.*

RIGHT: *Plate 30 The Aero chocolate-like cut surface of the liver that results from* Clostridium novyi *infection.*

after an hour if necessary). In practice, once brain oedema has occurred treatment is virtually impossible. In such cases, losses can be limited by removing the water supply and gradually rehydrating the normal pigs.

Organophosphorus Poisoning

Organophosphates are widely used as insecticides and have an accumulative effect as a neurotoxin (acute toxaemia has rarely been seen in pigs and produces vomiting and salivation). Contamination of feeding stuffs has been associated with posterior paralysis in sows as a result of degenerative changes in the spinal cord. In one outbreak in the UK in the late 1980s, problems occurred in weaned sows that had been receiving high levels of contaminated feed during lactation. The contamination occurred as a result of carriage of straights (grain screenings) in the hold of a ship that had previously been treated with organophosphate insecticide, but had not been washed out.

Treatment
The paralysis is permanent and humane destruction essential.

Nitrite Poisoning

Nitrates are widely distributed in the agricultural environment and are a major component of slurry. They are also widely used as non-organic fertilizers. Under the effects of certain microbial activity, nitrates are converted to nitrites. This process can also occur in the intestine. Nitrite binds with haemoglobin – the oxygen-carrying protein contained in the red blood cells – to produce methaemoglobin, which cannot carry oxygen. This, in effect, leads to internal asphyxiation or anoxia.

Clinical signs include rapid breathing and heart rate, salivation, dilated pupils and convulsions. Death is often associated with obvious cyanosis (blue discoloration) of the extremities. On post-mortem examination, the carcass is typically discoloured brown, but care should be taken as the gut may contain nitrogen dioxide gas.

Prevention
In the indoor piggery, nitrite poisoning is usually the result of poor ventilation, so that the animals have access to condensed water, or availability of dirty water such as roof drainage. Puddling of water outdoors and heavy algal contamination of outdoor water troughs can also encourage nitrite formulation. A clean water supply will go a long way to avoiding problems.

MISCELLANEOUS CONDITIONS

Pantothenic Acid Deficiency

Pantothenic acid is part of the B group of vitamins and is essential for maintenance of nerve integrity. Deficiency of pantothenic acid leads to degeneration of peripheral nerves, with consequent loss of motor control. The circumstances in which such deficiency occurs are usually feed errors or omissions – pantothenic acid would normally be included in a standard vitamin/mineral supplement. A failure to include the supplement in home-mixed rations is occasionally seen and may also occur where waste feeding is practised.

The classic description of pantothenic acid deficiency is one of 'goose-stepping' growing pigs. However, in practice it presents with a range of signs, including abnormal gait, splay-leg, weakness, swaying hind end and abnormal posture. There is no raised temperature. (*See* Figs 87 and 88.)

Treatment
Treatment with multivitamin injection containing D-pantothol can give a good response in mildly affected animals over a period of two to three weeks, but advanced cases require euthanasia.

PMWS/PDNS Neuropathy

The twin conditions of post-weaning multisystemic wasting syndrome (PMWS) and porcine dermatitis nephropathy syndrome (PDNS) are described in Chapters 7 and 10. It is, however, necessary to highlight the nervous manifestations of these complex diseases, which have not yet been fully investigated.

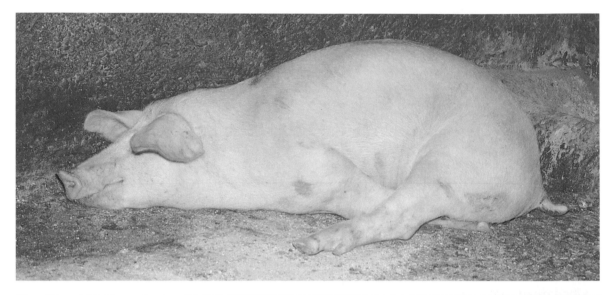

Figs 87 and 88 Pantothenic acid deficiency leading to loss of muscle control.

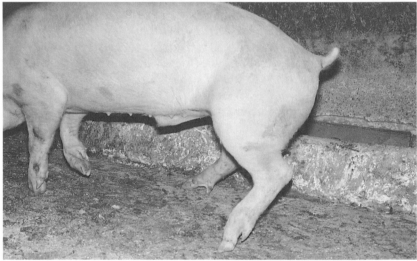

While it is unclear as to the pathology involved, in a small proportion of PMWS cases incoordination, ataxia and convulsions are seen in individuals unaffected with secondary disease (for example, Glasser's disease). Equally, a very small proportion of PDNS cases develop a progressive uncontrolled muscle tremor that ultimately leads to overt shaking, such that the pig is unable to eat or drink. Most cases will die or will be destroyed humanely. Again, it is unclear as to the precise pathology, but the clinical signs suggest that a progressive demyelination may be occurring. If so, it can be speculated that this is immune-mediated, given the perceived pathogenesis of PDNS as a whole.

In practice, ailments affecting the nervous system in the pig can be hard to differentiate and individual neurological examination is difficult in field conditions. With the pet pig, neurological disease can be dealt with in exactly the same way as would apply to a dog or a cat. In the farm situation, however, post-mortem examination is the most useful diagnostic tool.

CHAPTER NINE

Locomotor Disease and Lameness

There is considerable clinical overlap between lameness (the abnormal weight-bearing or gait changes that occur as a result of muscular-skeletal abnormalities) and loss of locomotor function as a result of abnormality of the nerve supply to the muscles. The latter is dealt with in Chapter 8, and it will be necessary for the reader to refer to that chapter as we work through localized conditions of the limbs that cause gait abnormality.

Alterations to the gait can arise as a result of pain somewhere in the limb (foot, bone, joint, tendon, ligament or muscle), or as a result of physical swelling that can interfere with the free movement of a joint, in which case pain is not necessarily involved. In continuing the general theme of this book, the aim of this chapter is to describe the various conditions seen in the different age groups.

Young Piglet Locomotor Problems

- Joint ill/polyarthritis – *see* pages 99–100.
- Splay-leg – *see* page 34.
- Congenital tremor – *see* page 36.
- Foot damage and abrasion – *see* page 103.
- Scuffed knees – *see* page 129.
- Congenital thick forelegs – *see* page 104.
- Arthrogryposis – *see* page 32.
- Injection damage – *see* page 104.
- Pietrain creeper syndrome – *see* page 104.

Inevitably, there will be conditions that occur in a range of ages and these will be explained.

YOUNG PIGLETS

The wide range of locomotor problems seen in the neonatal and young piglet are listed in the box below. A number of these conditions are dealt with elsewhere, while this chapter considers only some of the most common abnormalities.

Joint Ill

This is the colloquial term applied to infected joints (arthritis) in the pre-weaned pig and can affect one or more joints. The disease may be caused by specific infectious agents or by opportunist bacteria that gain entry to the joint via the bloodstream. The most common bacteria found in single-joint arthritis include staphylococci, streptococci, *E. coli* and *Arcanobacterium pyogenes* (formerly *Actinomyces pyogenes*), which are acquired from the environment or the skin of the piglet.

The start point for the onset of arthritis is bacteria gaining access to the bloodstream of the piglet to set up a bacteriaemia. Adequate colostrum intake will prevent bacteriaemia becoming established and, as such, wherever problems of joint ill occur, colostrum management should be reviewed. The bacteria gain entry by any breach of the integument (surface structures), including the navel in the first twelve hours, tail-dock wound, fight wounds, castration wounds, foot damage, teeth clipping and dirty injection technique. In addition, some specific organisms, such as *Streptococcus suis* and *Haemophilus parasuis*, can colonize and penetrate the tonsil, not requiring an artificial breach to do so.

The clinical presentation of joint ill will depend upon the number of joints affected. In the simple, single-joint arthritis, the pig may continue to suckle properly and, initially at least, not show any loss of condition. An uneven amount of weight will be placed on the affected limb, so that the pig shows anything from a mild limp to complete failure to bear its weight. Signs can be seen from two or three days of age, although peak incidence occurs in the second week of life. The piglet may have a raised temperature (40°C/104°F or above), be reluctant to leave the creep area and may squeal in pain on handling. Swelling and heat in the affected joint may also be evident, most readily seen in hocks, knees, elbows and stifles (*see* Fig. 89).

The consequences of joint ill can be serious. First, mobility is compromised, thus rendering the piglet far more susceptible to trampling, crushing or overlaying by the sow. Second, if left untreated, the arthritis will progress to a purulent form which, ultimately, will burst out of the joint as an abscess. This degree of joint damage is so severe as to require the humane destruction of the piglet.

Treatment
If joint ill is detected early, use of aggressive antimicrobial treatment can give good response. The choice of antibiotics will depend

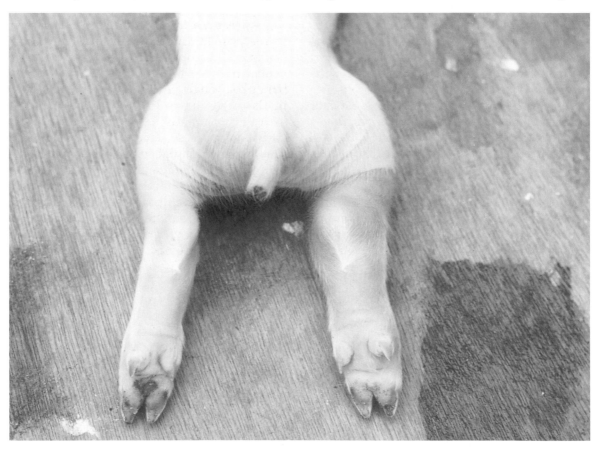

Fig. 89 Severe hind limb swelling associated with joint ill.

upon farm experience and cultures taken from affected joints (either at post-mortem examination or by aspiration from the joints). Synthetic penicillins (such as amoxycillin) and lincomycin are often the medicine of choice owing to their spectrum of activity and good penetration of the joint. It is vital, however, that treatment is given for a prolonged period – at least five days. Failure to treat for long enough may lead to an initial apparent recovery followed by relapse. In many cases, the relapse may not occur until after weaning, by which time it is often forgotten whether the pig had been an earlier case of joint ill or not.

Prevention
Prevention of joint ill depends upon ensuring adequate colostrum intake (discussed in Chapter 3) and minimizing the risk of bacteria gaining entry to the bloodstream. Hygiene and technique are the key.

Sows should enter cleaned and disinfected farrowing accommodation no more than seven days prior to expected farrowing (during periods longer than a week, the level of contamination by the sow rather undoes the effect of cleaning and disinfecting). All solid faeces should be removed from the farrowing pen when produced (it rarely falls through the small slatted area).

At birth, copious amounts of clean bedding will reduce faecal contamination (shredded paper works well on slatted floors). The wet navel should be dipped with iodine – this is more effective than spraying, as it ensures that the open wound of the navel is treated rather than the base of the navel.

Tail docking (discussed in Chapter 3) is normally performed in the first three days of life. A clean technique is essential and, in particular, the same clippers used to remove teeth (*see* below) must not be used for the tail (the mouth harbours many bacteria). Ideally, some form of thermocauterization should be used to dock tails, as this seals the wound and prevents infection. Where clippers are used and bleeding results, the docked tail should be dipped in iodine.

Obviously, aseptic techniques should be used for injections (with a change of needle between each litter – for example, when administering iron treatments) and for castration. In the latter case, it is vital that postoperative hygiene is maintained to prevent wound contamination.

The requirements and techniques for teeth clipping are discussed in Chapter 3, but in terms of hygiene the key features are:

1. The mouth becomes heavily contaminated with bacteria that are acquired from the vagina of the sow during the birth process, from the teat of the sow during early suckling or from the pen floor.
2. If the teeth shatter (as opposed to a smooth cut close to the gum) this will open up a route into the bloodstream and allow the primary bacteriaemia to occur. Teeth clipping does not lead to joint ill per se; rather, it is poor technique that causes the condition.

Streptococcus suis Type 14 (SS14)
In the early 1990s in the UK and parts of Europe, an apparently new disease was described, quite distinct from the acute post-weaning meningitis seen as a result of *Streptococcus suis* type II infection (*see* Chapter 8). Many stockmen initially confused it with meningitis, which is a rare finding with *S. suis* type 14, although it does occasionally occur as a complication. Primarily affecting pigs two to three weeks of age (but also found in older pigs up to three months of age), *S. suis* type 14 causes a very severe polyarthritis. The key features of this disease are as follows:

1. Very dramatic, sudden onset affecting several or all pigs in a litter.
2. The piglets show intense pain.
3. Many piglets simply lay about, gently moving their legs while emitting a dull squeal.

Up to 50 per cent of all piglets can be affected and the disease course within a herd can last for more than a year. However, individual piglet

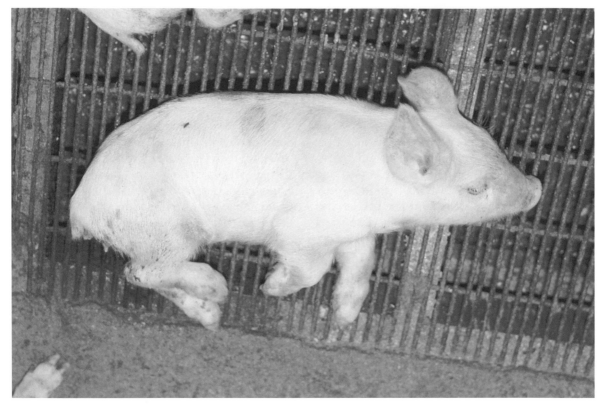

Fig. 90 Streptococcus suis *type 14 infection, causing very painful polyarthritis (joint ill).*

response to treatment with simple penicillin is dramatic and curative – a single treatment will often suffice.

The disease appears to be spread by stock introduced into a farm previously free from infection. Features that influence both the incidence and the persistence of the disease include high gilt replacement rates, large farrowing groups within the same air space, and continually occupied farrowing rooms. It has been postulated that a few gilts act as the reservoir of infection (which is probably excreted by the tonsils and, thus, spread in the air), and colostral protection seems poor or short-lived. The large number of sows in a farrowing room is presumed to create a higher infective dose for the litters. As a general rule, while the disease is seen in the outdoor environment with sows farrowing in individual arcs, the incidence is much higher indoors in large rooms.

Prevention
Treatment of sows prior to farrowing and during lactation is highly effective at reducing the excretion of bacteria and, thus, at reducing the incidence of clinical disease. This can be achieved in one of three ways:

1. Sow feed medication included at source, using either penicillin or potentiated sulphonamides. The difficulty arising here is setting the dose rate, as sow daily feed intake varies from as little as 1kg (2lb 3oz) on the day of farrowing up to a maximum of 10kg (22lb) in late lactation.
2. Individual sow treatment by 'top dressing' a daily dose of antibiotics (again, penicillin or potentiated sulphonamides are most effective) onto the feed. In this way, a fixed daily dose can be given to each sow and effective control can be achieved by treating daily

from entry to the farrowing house up to farrowing, and, thereafter, treating on alternate days. Unfortunately, under EU medicine laws, most in-feed antibiotics (pre-mixes) are licensed only for 'incorporation' into feed and, thus, the application by top dressing is illegal. The third method may therefore be more suitable.

3. The same daily dose effect as above can be achieved using water-soluble antibiotic preparations made up as a concentrate and added onto the feed in the same way as top dressing. If carried out under veterinary guidance, this technique does not fall foul of medicine regulations so long as withdrawal periods are sufficient before slaughter.

As an alternative to treating sows to prevent excretion of bacteria, piglets can be treated by injection at three, ten and seventeen days with long-acting penicillin or ceftiofur. This is equally effective but far more labour intensive, so the comparative costs of the different treatments must be assessed.

It should be noted that, while an outbreak of *S. suis* type 14 infection can persist in a herd for a prolonged period in many farms, the disease usually simply disappears in a few months. Thus, in all cases where a preventative programme has been put in place, its continuing necessity should be tested periodically by leaving some sows/litters untreated to see if disease returns.

Haemophilus parasuis

Infection with *Haemophilus parasuis* can occur in a similar way to *Streptococcus suis* type 14, but most commonly results in coughing and respiratory disease in pigs ten or more days old and so is described in more detail in Chapter 7. Occasionally, piglets will develop polyarthritis or meningitis before weaning due to *Haemophilus parasuis* infection, but, unlike *S. suis* type 14, there is a very poor response to treatment in affected piglets.

Prevention

Prevention of disease can be effected in the same way as with *S. suis* type 14, although here individual piglet injection appears to give better results than medicating sows, suggesting that other piglets are a more significant source of infection than sows.

Foot Damage and Abrasions

Piglets are born into a wide range of environments in which floor type in particular is highly variable. A suitable floor type is one that gives sufficient grip without being abrasive, is non-damaging, is cleanable and clean, is warm and is affordable. Inevitably, these requirements lead to compromise, and many piglets

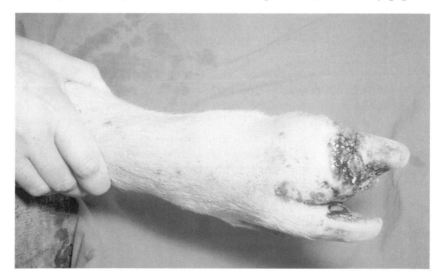

Fig. 91 Severe lameness in the baby pig results from infection through damaged feet.

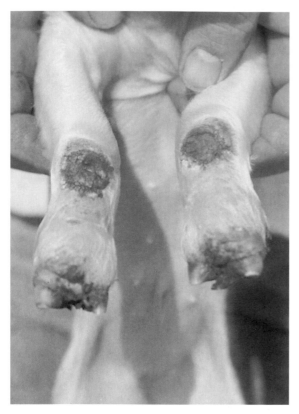

Fig. 92 Scuffed knees are usually a sign of bad floors.

are born onto floors that are either slippery (risking splay-leg), abrasive (causing bruising to feet, erosion of claws and abrasion to knees) or damaging (causing entrapment of feet, abrasion of the coronary band and removal of claws). In all these cases, the physical damage leads to lameness in itself, and it can also lead on to secondary infection and either local abscessation or haematogenous spread.

Prevention
Feet damage to piglets is seen least often in deep-bedded straw systems but, unfortunately, these may have other disadvantages, such as higher contamination levels, wet flooring and high labour requirements. Conversely, some forms of slats (for example, concrete slats and expanded metal sheets) are totally unsuitable for newborn piglets. Plastic-coated

wire floors may give the best compromise and, while expensive, this material does tend to be very long-lasting.

Injection Damage
Lameness can result from muscle or nerve damage to the piglet as a result of physical injury caused by high-volume injection into small muscle masses. Injections of 2ml doses of, for example, vaccines and iron preparations into the ham (back of the back leg) provide a high risk of damaging the muscle (which happens to be one of the most valuable parts of the carcass) or the sciatic nerve, which runs down the back of the thigh bone (femur).

Prevention
It is always preferable to inject piglets in the muscles of the neck rather than the ham and, where small doses are available (especially with iron injections) these are preferred. Damage can be particularly severe in PRRS-affected piglets. Aseptic technique is also essential to prevent infection and abscess formation at the site of injection.

Congenital Thick Forelegs
This is an inherited condition governed by an autosomal recessive gene and is seen most often in Landrace piglets (*see* Fig. 23). The thickening of the lower forelimbs impedes movement, rendering the piglet very vulnerable to crushing. Provided the piglet can suckle and secondary infection does not occur, approximately 30 per cent of cases can recover and the thickened legs will resolve.

Prevention
In order to prevent the continuation of this condition in future generations, animals with thick forelegs should not be used for breeding.

Piertran Creeper Syndrome
This is an extremely rare progressive muscle degenerative disease (myopathy), of which mild forms may occur in the Landrace breed. It is likely to be an inherited condition. Initial muscle trembling and tiptoed gait ultimately give

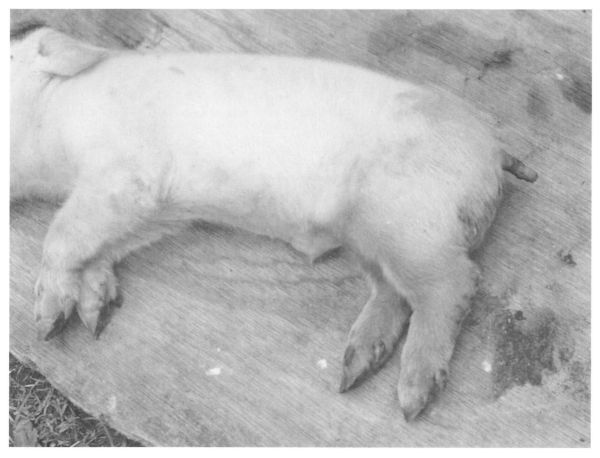

Fig. 93 Bruising of the leg muscle as a result of injection can be severe in pigs affected with PRRS.

way to weakness and recumbency, while the animal remains appetant, alert and growing.

Treatment
There is no cure and humane destruction is necessary.

GROWING PIGS

Infectious Arthritis
Individual joint-infected arthritis is a common sporadic disease in pigs aged from four to twenty-four weeks of age. As with infection in the baby piglet, opportunist bacteria gain entry to the bloodstream and spread to the joints. The primary causes of such infection are as follows:

1. Residual joint infection in the younger piglet following inadequate treatment.
2. Penetration of wounds and, in particular, foot injuries.
3. Infection secondary to tail-biting – this is the most common form of sporadic arthritis in finishing pigs.
4. Secondary to *Streptococcus suis* infection, especially types II and 14.

Treatment
Once infection has got into the joint, abscessation will occur and ultimately this may burst out. Treatment of such well-developed lesions is hopeless and, as such, affected animals are not suitable for human consumption. On-farm humane destruction is required.

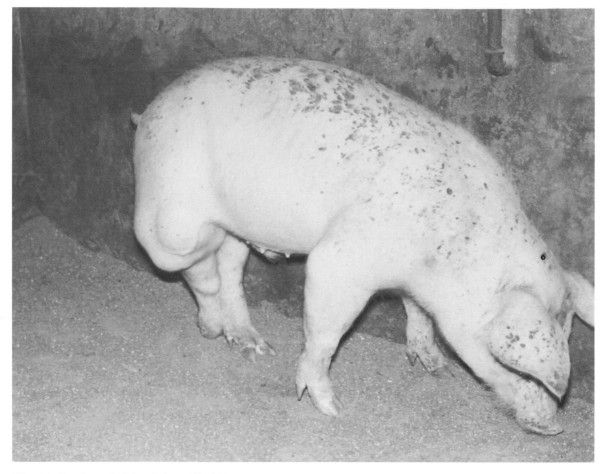

Fig. 94 Septic arthritis of the stifle joint.

Detection and treatment in early cases may be more successful but, as with infection in baby piglets, a prolonged treatment of at least five days is often needed.

Mycoplasma hyosynoviae Infection

Infection and disease associated with *Mycoplasma hyosynoviae* infection can affect any pigs from 25kg (55lb) up to the young adult. There is a sudden onset of lameness, often affecting two or more limbs. If the hind legs are affected, the pig may dog-sit and shuffle about. In less severe cases, muscle trembling will be seen as the pig struggles to rise. When moved, an affected pig will walk with a stiff, awkward gait and may collapse on its back end. If the front legs are affected, the pig will move with a very stiff gait and obviously be in pain. Severely affected pigs may grind their teeth and be recumbent. A mild pyrexia may also be present, probably secondary to pain rather than infection.

The disease is more common in straw-based systems and, in particular, those with a scrape-through dunging passage. The causative organism is capable of surviving in moist conditions for up to four weeks and, once present, can lead to a progressive problem – more disease leads to greater *Mycoplasma* excretion, providing a higher dose to infect young following animals. In the older growing pig, and particularly replacement gilts, a second bout of lameness can occur following transportation, remixing, change of diet and puberty. The higher incidence of disease in replacement gilts (compared to boars) suggests a hormonal component to the relapse, although trauma as a result of oestrus females riding each other cannot be ruled out.

Diagnosis can be difficult. Serology can be confusing in that seropositive (in other words, 'immune') gilts can still show clinical disease, and the organism is also very hard to culture. In addition, the disease often occurs in conjunction with osteochondrosis (*see* below). *Mycoplasma hyosynoviae* does not cause osteoarthritic damage and, as such, there is no lasting lameness unless osteochondrosis is also involved. Response to treatment is often regarded as confirmation of a clinical diagnosis.

Treatment
In uncomplicated *M. hyosynoviae* infection, rapid response is seen to tiamulin or lincomycin therapy. Often the animal is completely sound within twenty-four hours, although a failure to provide follow-up treatment (a three-day

course) may lead to a relapse between three and five days later. (Care should also be taken to prevent ionophore toxicity – *see* page 110.)

Erysipelas
Infection with *Erysipelothrix rhusiopathiae* in pigs causes a wide range of clinical signs, including skin lesions (*see* Chapter 10), sudden death and reproductive failure (*see* Chapter 1). In the acute stages of erysipelas (known as 'diamonds'), the legs may be stiff and the animal reluctant to walk. This is a feature of all septicaemic disease but does not necessarily indicate the presence of arthritis; it may simply reflect muscle pain.

Lameness due to arthritis caused by erysipelas is a chronic debilitating disease that results from a type III hypersensitivity (allergic) reaction to the initial infection – in other words, it is a disease of the recovery phase. It can also occur in partially immune animals, which means that the preceding typical signs of erysipelas (the diamond-shaped skin lesions

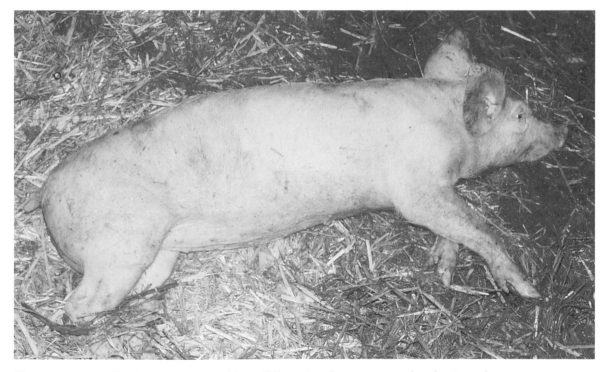

Fig. 95 It is usually clinically impossible to differentiate between osteochondrosis and acute Mycoplasma *arthritis.*

described in Chapter 10) may not be seen. The lameness is severe and progressive, with pigs adopting a hunched back and very stiff legs. In the adult it may be difficult to differentiate clinically between erysipelas arthritis and chronic mild osteochondrosis, although the occurrence of associated osteoarthritis is obvious at post-mortem. Cultures from affected joints, which may be swollen, hard or fluid-filled, will often be sterile and diagnosis must be made on a herd basis by serology or on post-mortem by histopathology. It may be possible to detect high antibody levels to erysipelas in the joint fluid.

Treatment
Treatment in the early stages of lameness is more effective if cortisone or non-steroidal anti-inflammatories are used in conjunction with penicillin. Advanced cases require euthanasia.

Prevention and Control
Vaccination for erysipelas will not protect against this form of the disease per se (because it is an immune-mediated disease), but a herd vaccine programme used over a period of time will reduce the burden of infection in the environment and, as such, will help slowly to reduce

lameness. Erysipelas has become increasingly common in the UK as more pigs are grown on in straw-based systems that are accessible to both rodents and birds. The disease is therefore a major risk to future breeding stock, which are often reared under such conditions.

Osteochondrosis
The joint surfaces of the bones are covered with a cushion of cartilage. Furthermore, the bones grow from cartilaginous growth plates (called epiphyseal plates) close to the tips of the bone. Defects in cartilage are termed osteochondrosis and have been shown to be present microscopically in 100 per cent of pigs at one day of age in all breed types, including wild boar.

In some pigs, this precursor damage can lead to severe abnormality of the joint as the pig grows. The cartilage may crack, lift, erode or split, exposing underlying bone. The grinding of bone against bone is extremely painful and a severe lameness results, often affecting several joints. However, deformity of the cartilage in itself is not painful and many pigs at slaughter weight (100kg/220lb live weight) can be seen to have abnormal joint cartilage without having been lame (*see* Plate 7). The highly variable gaits of growing pigs may be related more to this deformity than to pain. Defects in the cartilage of the growth plates can also lead to spontaneous separation of the tip of the bone (pathological fractures); this is discussed in greater detail under the heading 'Fractures and Injuries' below.

Overt clinical disease associated with osteochondrosis can be seen in pigs above 40kg (90lb) through to adults, and the pathogenesis and epidemiology appear particularly complex. It is possible here only to highlight briefly some of the management factors that appear to be associated with clinical disease:

1. Exercise during the young growing phase – large amounts of space in which young pigs can run around, particularly if they slip, seems to bring on osteochondritic damage.
2. Overcrowding/excessive stocking rates in young growing pigs (30–60kg/65–130lb) can

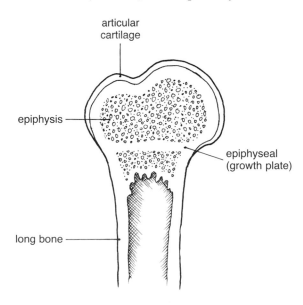

Fig. 96 Structure of the end of a long bone.

articular cartilage

epiphysis

epiphyseal (growth plate)

long bone

trigger osteochondrosis in older animals (around 100kg/220lb).

3. Abnormal calcium/phosphorus ration in diets.
4. Acidic diets and metabolic acidosis.
5. Growth that is too fast and heavy muscling. (Animals subjected to bovine growth hormone treatment or the result of genetic modification regimes have been crippled with osteochondritic arthritis and so such programmes have largely been abandoned.)
6. Breed type – Landrace in particular seem to be affected.
7. Slippery floors.

The clinical presentation of osteochondrosis can be highly variable. As explained above, in mild cases in growing pigs intended for slaughter the signs may be so vague and insignificant that no notice is taken. However, similar signs in gilts destined for breeding will lead to rejection on the grounds of conformation, lameness or simply the knowledge that an abnormal gait is likely to result in overt lameness as the gilt approaches breeding (125kg/275lb live weight). In more severe cases, clinical lameness may be evident: there may be difficulty in rising, particularly on the hind end (compare with *Mycoplasma* arthritis on page 106); there may be a stilled gait with hunched back; or the animal may be totally recumbent. There will be no pyrexia.

Treatment
Once the damage has occurred it is practically irresolvable and slaughter – either as a casualty animal or on-farm euthanasia – is appropriate.

Prevention and Control
Control of the condition lies in being able to identify the specific trigger factors and then correcting them. If these relate to stocking density and space provision, it is relatively easy to prevent the problem from occurring. Where it is simply the result of heavily muscled fast-growing pigs in commercial conditions, control can be very difficult and costly.

Fractures and Injuries

Spontaneous fractures are common sporadic features of modern pig-keeping. The fast growth and very young, soft bones renders pigs susceptible to fracture as a result of slipping, banging against walls and potholes or riding each other. The areas most commonly affected are the shoulder (usually as a result of banging against a vertical support) and the upper hind legs. In the latter case, the main long bone (femur) may fracture at the tip where it forms the hip joint. The anatomy of this joint is such that, if the legs splay out sideways (the 'splits'), the greater trochanter can act as a pivot against the pelvis and the head of the femur will break off either at its base (a true fracture) or at the epiphyseal plate if osteochondritic changes are significant (epiphysiolysis).

Occasionally, outbreaks of fractures will occur in young growing pigs around 30kg/65lb in weight. These appear to be associated with previous infectious damage (for example, *Streptococcus suis* type 14) to the epiphyseal plate – when the pigs are released into open spaces such as large straw yards, the physical exertion leads to separation of the growth plates in the lower tibia (above the hock).

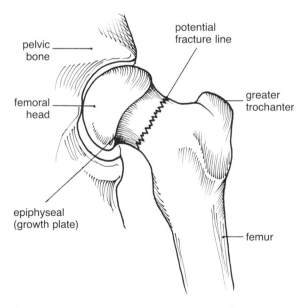

Fig. 97 Diagramatic representation of the pig hip joint.

Treatment

In all these cases, treatment is not practical in the commercial environment and humane destruction is appropriate. In the pet pig, fracture repairs can be effected in exactly the same way as with a dog; readers are referred to standard orthopaedic texts.

Ionophore Toxicity

Ionophores are chemicals used in the poultry industry as coccidiostats and in the pig industry as growth promoters. As of January 2006, their use in the EU is banned. Ionophores are toxic if used to excess, and this toxicity is exacerbated when they are combined with tiamulin or valnemulin; these products must therefore not be used in conjunction in feed. However, the greatest risk of toxicity results from therapeutic treatment of growing pigs with tiamulin (for example, by injection for *Mycoplasma* arthritis treatment or via water for swine dysentery treatment) when the diet, unknowingly, contains salinomycin or some other ionophore.

Toxic levels of ionophores have an effect on the muscles, such that the pig is recumbent or off its back legs. Some may even be found dead. The muscles may be trembling, temperatures will be in the region of 40–41°C (104–106°F), respiratory rates are raised and laboured breathing will be evident. Milder cases may simply be ataxic (wobbly on their legs). The muscle masses tend to be hard and the pigs emit a distinctive squealing noise, exacerbated on handling, that is different to any other sound the author has heard from pigs. On post-mortem examination, muscle tissue is pale but otherwise no gross lesions are visible (acute myopathy can be confirmed on histopathological examination).

Treatment

The condition appears to be progressive, even after removal of medicated feed, and recovery of anything but the mildest cases is rare. Ionophore toxicity in sheep is known to have the effect of totally depleting circulating vitamin E levels, but as treatment with injectable vitamin E gives a very poor response in pigs

this would suggest that the condition results in differing consequences in these animals.

Other Toxicities

Selenium

Selenium is an essential trace element and is part of the antioxidant system, working in conjunction with vitamin E. Supplementary levels are included in diets, but occasionally errors occur and excess may be included. Acute toxicity is associated with leg weakness, ataxia, trembling of the muscles, collapse and death. Damage to the brain can be detected at postmortem examination. Chronic (in other words, long-term build-up) toxicity due to selenium leads to hair loss and cracking/separation of the hoof. Piglets born to sows receiving excess selenium not only have a raised stillbirth level but are born with characteristic haemorrhages on the soles and walls of the claws.

Removal of excess selenium can lead to recovery over a prolonged period of six to eight weeks. Plants of the *Astragalus* genus (for example, milkvetch) contain high levels of selenium and, as such, access to them should be restricted.

Zinc

Zinc is another micronutrient essential for normal body function. In addition, zinc oxide is widely used in weaned pigs as a preventative treatment for post-weaning scouring. Zinc oxide is totally insoluble, is restricted to the gut and, even though it is fed at levels that supply 2,500ppm or more of zinc, it is not toxic. Levels of 2,000ppm of soluble zinc (as zinc sulphate, zinc carbonate and so on) are, however, highly toxic to pigs, causing growth depression, muscular haemorrhage and arthritis (as a result of haemorrhage in joints). Thus, a problem of zinc toxicity will present as rather more complex than simple lameness.

Lime Burn

Hydrated lime is used as a final disinfectant in concrete buildings, the very high pH killing most microbes, including those present in organic matter such as faeces. It is widely used in straw yards, where washing out is often less than thorough.

The chemical reaction of lime and water takes three to four days to complete, and if pigs are placed in pens prior to this time scalding can occur. In mild forms, such scalding can cause ulcers to the coronary band and snout without lameness (as would occur with foot and mouth disease and swine vesicular disease). However, rarely the effect may be so severe that the soft horn of the foot is scorched – particularly if the pigs have been outdoors or on deep straw, such that the sole and heel are very soft. In these cases, pigs will appear to walk on tiptoe, have a very stilted gait and be reluctant to move. Ulcers on the ventral body may be evident where pigs have been recumbent.

The condition will pass with time as the lime cures and the scalding effect passes. Removal to deep straw will accelerate recovery. Ulceration of the foot could occur in particularly severe cases and, in these, recovery will be delayed.

ADULTS

Lameness is a major reason for both premature culling and on-farm euthanasia in breeding sows, and on many indoor commercial pig farms up to 6 per cent of the sow population may be destroyed each year owing to this condition. The major causes of such lameness are septic laminitis (bush foot), leg weakness, fractures, spinal lesions and multiple degenerative arthritis. Many of the problems seen in sows can be traced back to joint damage during the growing stages, either as a result of infection (for example, erysipelas) or degenerative joint disease (osteochondrosis). Boars can be affected with any of the conditions described below.

Septic Laminitis

Bush foot is a common condition of the pig and results from infection gaining entry through cracks in the sole or wall of the claw. The types of lesions seen are not as well characterized as those in the dairy cow, and because of the reduced mobility of sows the condition is often not detected until swelling and abscessation are evident above the coronary band. Rupture of the abscess will be evident, either on the side of the claw or in the inter-digital space. The sow will be severely lame and resistant to handling of the foot. The foot will be hot and painful; if investigated, this can frequently be detected in a lame sow before swelling is evident.

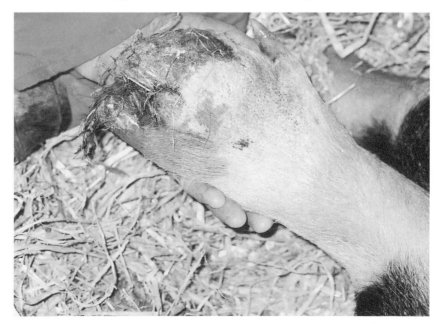

Fig. 98 Septic laminitis (bush foot), with purulent break-out at the coronary band.

Treatment and Prevention

The key to treatment is to drain the pus, which can be done either by applying a poultice or by simple debridement of tissue and washing. Follow-up treatment with antibiotics (particularly lincomycin) and non-steroidal anti-inflammatory painkillers can be highly successful. However, to treat a swollen foot solely with antibiotics is a case of too little too late and response is often poor.

Bush foot results from damage to the claw and subsequent contamination. The quality of the floor therefore has a major role to play – rough abrasive floors and broken slats are particularly significant. Efforts to improve horn quality by foot bathing (for example, in copper sulphate or formalin) have proved to be of dubious value and are complicated by the tendency of sows to try to drink it! Horn integrity does, however, seem to improve with supplementary biotin in the diet, which can help reduce the incidence of cracking and subsequent infection (*see* below).

Overgrown Claws

Severe overgrowth of claws results from the high-protein ration fed to sows, particularly during lactation, coupled with lack of exercise and hence a reduced wearing down of the claws. Moreover, some breed types may have dropped pasterns, which tend to allow horn overgrowth (to some extent, this occurs in many sows as they age).

Severe claw overgrowth can lead to difficulties in walking and a tendency for the legs to slip from under the sow, thereby putting her at risk from further injury. Overgrown claws are also prone to breaking off and becoming infected, or can simply crack so that bush foot is allowed to develop. The problem is particularly prevalent in confined conditions and may also be seen in association with osteochondrosis.

Treatment

When the condition is severe, trimming or even sanding of the claw to restore the normal shape can be worthwhile and prolong the working life of the sow.

Fractures

In the same way that spontaneous fractures occur in growing pigs (*see* page 109), the sow is particularly vulnerable to hip damage. Separation of the head of the femur (epiphysiolysis) through the growth plate can occur at any time up until closure, which occurs between 3 and 3½ years of age. It is a sudden-onset total limb lameness and can be bilateral, leading to a dog-sitting position. The injury has its roots in prior osteochondritic changes.

Apophysiolysis is a similar condition that is clinically indistinguishable from epiphysiolysis.

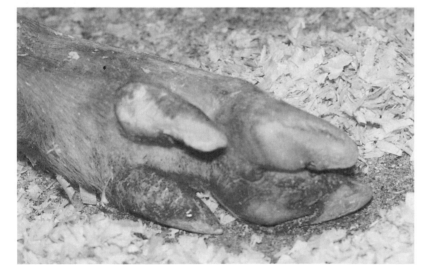

Fig. 99 Overgrowth of claws can be both a cause of problems and a result of lameness (particularly joint disease).

Here, the epiphysis of the pelvis (tuber ischium) is pulled off by the muscle mass supporting the limb. In both cases, the injury may be precipitated by slipping (floor quality is therefore critical) or bullying and riding. Injury is particularly likely when weaned sows are grouped together prior to service.

Spontaneous long-bone fractures can occur in weaned sows as a result of osteoporosis, the drain on calcium and phosphorous reserves that occurs during lactation. Here, the bones become decalcified and brittle, and are therefore more susceptible to fracture. Gilts are particularly vulnerable to the calcium drain, especially if they rear a large litter, and once the piglets are weaned they are vulnerable to any of the conditions mentioned above, not least epiphysiolysis. Inadequate nutrition during lactation is common in gilts and forms part of the 'second litter drop' syndrome.

Prevention
Ensuring that gilts are bred only when old enough (at least seven months) and big enough (120kg/265lb-plus live weight), using only properly formulated and balanced diets and restricting lactation lengths goes a long way to reducing the risks of osteoporosis and hence related injury.

Posterior Paresis
Partial paralysis of the back legs (posterior paresis) is a common clinical presentation in both the gilt and sow, and can be the result of a number of causes:

1. Epiphysiolysis.
2. Apophysiolysis.
3. Spinal abscess.
4. Adductor muscle tear.
5. Fracture of the femur or femoral head.
6. Viral encephalitis (for example, caused by Aujeszky's disease or Talfan).
7. Chronic organophosphate poisoning.
8. Heavy metal poisoning (particularly mercury).
9. Pigweed (*Amaranthus*) poisoning.
10. Organic arsenical poisoning.

Treatment
The treatment given will depend on diagnosing the cause of paralysis.

Biotin Responsive Lameness
Biotin is one of the group of B vitamins, a deficiency of which in sows is associated with infertility and specific breaches in the integrity of the horn of the foot such that horizontal lesions (cracks) are seen across it. Such conditions are rare and respond to supplementary biotin in the diet, although in affected sows the response can take six months to be seen owing to the slow growth of horn. Biotin responsive lameness is often, but not exclusively, reported in outdoor/free-range sows.

Treatment
Supplementary biotin added at a rate of 400mg per tonne as d-biotin can provide a clinical response to lameness and reduce the incidence of bush foot. It is particularly effective in situations where the classic signs of biotin deficiency are absent.

Laminitis
Inflammation of the lamina, which attaches the horn to the toe, is well documented in the dairy cow and is nutritional in origin. A similar situation has not been definitively described in sows but may exist, particularly in the outdoor system. Sporadic cases of laminitis in pigs do occur, usually as a result of haematogenous spread of bacterial toxins from a preceding metritis. The condition is, thus, seen in later lactation or post-weaning. The sow is reluctant to stand and even more reluctant to walk, but will respond to non-steroidal anti-inflammatory agents in combination with broad-spectrum antibiotics. The toes (claws) will be very hot to the touch, and in loose housed situations they may be very obviously dry despite wet conditions underfoot. In extreme cases, the whole claws may separate (thimbling), leaving raw, unprotected soft tissue exposed.

Treatment
Humane destruction is required immediately.

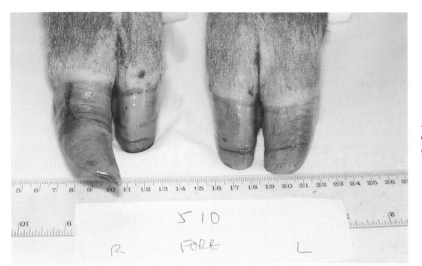

Fig. 100 Uneven horn growth evident as ridges is suggestive of laminitic damage.

Sunburn

Although it is not a true cause of lameness, severe sunburn in pigs can present in an alarming way that suggests the animal is lame. The pain and skin damage resulting from sunburn on the back causes the pig to try to relieve the cracking skin by altering the curvature of its spine. Affected animals will walk on their 'knees' (front-leg carpal joints) and the whole of the back will be dipped and curved concavely. When handled, the pig will tend to squeal in pain.

Treatment

Treatment with non-steroidal anti-inflammatories and emollient creams on the skin will reduce the pain and allow recovery after a few days. Light mineral oil, such as pig oil, can be used instead of creams, but the key to recovery is to remove the insult – in other words, the animal should be housed in the shade.

Exotic Diseases

As with respiratory disease, enteric disease and reproductive disease, the sudden onset of a number of signs, particularly among a wide age range of animals, should raise the possibility of a new infectious agent entering the herd. The 'exotic' diseases are particularly relevant in this respect.

In the context of lameness, both foot and mouth disease and swine vesicular disease must be considered. The two diseases are clinically indistinguishable, although because of the seriousness of foot and mouth, all suspected cases are assumed to be this until shown otherwise. Swine vesicular disease is a mild and transient disease of little welfare concern and of no economic issue in itself. Tell-tale signs of these diseases include vesicles that rupture to cause ulcers on the snout and feet (on the coronary band and inter-digital spaces). Affected pigs are acutely lame, reluctant to walk, inappetant and, in the early stages, have a raised temperature. Mortality in pigs is low (compared to cattle), but the pig is significant as a major generator of virus and, therefore, can be highly relevant in the spread of disease. In Europe and North America, state control programmes exist for foot and mouth, usually involving slaughter; elsewhere, vaccination may be practised.

Lameness in the pig represents one of the most significant attacks on the well-being of the animal, and is responsible for much pain and suffering as well as economic loss. Correct diagnosis and rapid, appropriate treatment, particularly including analgesics, are therefore vital if the welfare of the animal is to be addressed.

CHAPTER TEN

Skin Disease, Swellings and Superficial Injuries

In this chapter, we will look at the wide range of conditions that present with lesions evident on the surface of the pig. These may be either diseases specific to the skin or a sign of more widespread disease in the body, but they are particularly obvious and of diagnostic significance. In the modern, largely white breeds of pigs with very sparse hair coverage, defects or changes in the skin are often clear to see. The experienced clinician will be able to distinguish the specific causes purely by visual assessment of the lesion and the general demeanour of the pig, although laboratory tests may be appropriate to confirm a diagnosis.

The nature of group-housed pigs is such that injury as a result of fighting or vice constitutes some of the most common superficial lesions seen. However, specific infectious agents are implicated in some skin conditions and it is to these that we turn first.

BACTERIAL DISEASES

Exudative Epidermitis or Greasy Pig Disease

Probably the single most common significant disease affecting the skin of the pig is the multi-faceted condition that is usually called greasy pig disease (GPD) or exudative epidermitis (it is also known as marmite disease).

More accurately, this is a wide range of presentations resulting from infection of the skin (epidermis) with staphylococcal bacteria, specifically *Staphylococcus hyicus*.

S. hyicus is widely found within the pig population worldwide, living often as a normal commensal on the skin. A range of factors can lead to penetration of the skin by the bacteria, colonization of the living tissue and proliferation. Some of the key triggers for this are:

1. Fight wounds and any other injuries to the skin, including ulceration or abrasion on concrete floors, and damage to the lower limb and coronary band on slatted floors.
2. High levels of environmental contamination.
3. High humidity levels.
4. Low oxygen levels (poor ventilation).
5. Other skin disease such as pig pox, mange and ringworm.

Clinical Presentation
Depending on the age of the pig, the initial site of penetration and possibly the strain of bacteria involved, lesions will be highly variable. They may be:

1. Acute and extensive (*see* Plate 9).
2. Acute and ulcerative but localized (*see* Plate 10).
3. Extensive and chronic (*see* Plate 11).

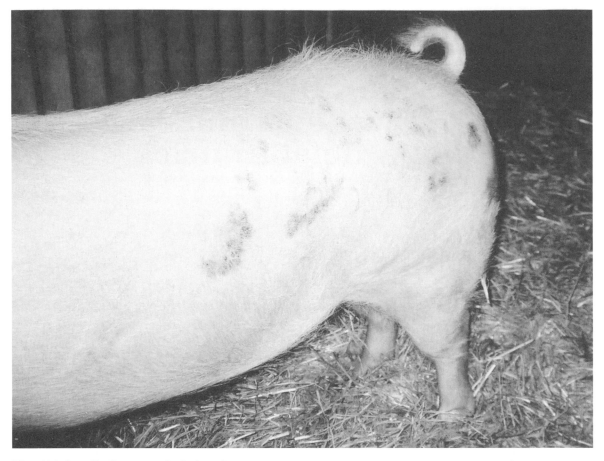

Fig. 101 Localized greasy pig lesions in a sow.

4. Localized and chronic (*see* Fig. 101).
5. Acute and localized around 'fighting areas', for example the shoulders (*see* Fig. 102).
6. On the tips of the ears, leading to secondary ear-tip necrosis as a result of penetrating thromboembolism (*see* Figs 103 and 104).
7. As a ring around the base of the tail, leading to tail necrosis (*see* Fig. 105).

One of the most significant features of *S. hyicus* infection in the pig is that it is non-pruritic (in other words, the pigs show no evidence of irritation), which is in marked contrast to the other very common skin condition of sarcoptic mange (*see* page 123).

Pigs as young as three to four days of age may be affected (with acute ulcerative skin disease or tail necrosis), but most typically the disease is seen in the following age groups:

1. Acute extensive disease – typically three to eight weeks of age, but can be seen down to five days of age.
2. Ulcerative disease – sporadic at any age, including sows, but can affect whole litters.
3. Extensive chronic disease – growers aged ten to twenty weeks.
4. Localized chronic lesions – adults.
5. Acute localized fight wounds – typically post-weaning.
6. Ear-tip necrosis – usually at eight to fifteen weeks of age, following initial lesions at six to seven weeks.
7. Tail necrosis – less than seven days of age.

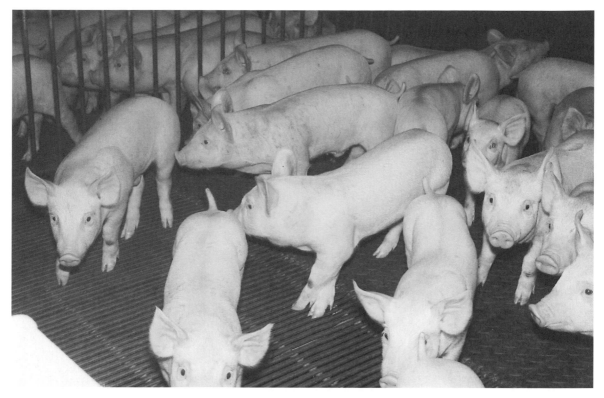

Fig. 102 Skin wounds caused by fighting after mixing at weaning are an important route of entry for bacterial infection.

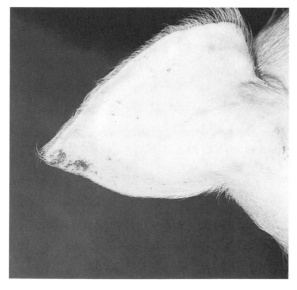

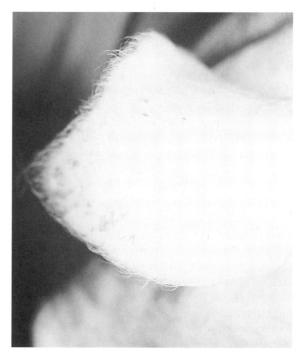

ABOVE: *Fig. 103 The initial lesion of ear-tip necrosis.*

Fig. 104 The advanced lesion of ear-tip necrosis.

117

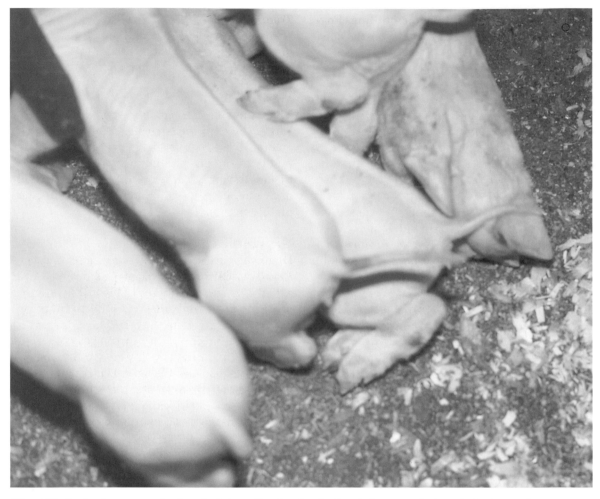

Fig. 105 Early damage to the head of the tail, allowing in Staphylococcus hyicus *infection and ultimately leading to tail necrosis.*

Treatment

In most cases, the bacteria remain localized in the skin and do not spread internally. However, disruption of the skin function can have a major effect on physiology and acute extensive disease can kill, particularly in the younger age groups.

Treatment is by a combination of fluid therapy (electrolytes, particularly in pigs younger than four weeks of age, antibiotics and skin sanitizers. The antibiotics of choice tend to be synthetic penicillin (for example, amoxycillin), lincomycin or cephalosporins (especially cephalexin), given parentally or orally. Topical treatment with novobiocin (a specific anti-staphylococcal agent included in some cattle intramammary preparations) mixed with light mineral oil is highly effective where available (this would most likely be off-licence use). Generally, treatment will be required for five to seven days to cure the active infection, although recovery of skin integrity can take up to a month. It is not usually necessary to treat pigs with chronic lesions, ear-tip necrosis or tail necrosis.

Washing pigs in soap or mild disinfectant is a useful adjunct to treatment for extensive acute disease, but if washing young pigs great

118

care must be exercised to avoid chilling. Fogging the atmosphere with disinfectant is used where outbreaks of acute disease are seen in weaners.

Prevention and Control
Prevention of disease-causing *Staphylococcus hyicus* infection relies upon good sanitation, the provision of fresh air and avoidance of skin damage from fighting or the environment. Keeping pigs separate, spraying them with deodorants and maintaining low stocking rates all help to reduce fighting and the attendant skin damage. Ear-tip necrosis can be very difficult to control but is of dubious economic significance, despite being extremely unsightly.

Careful introduction of new stock is needed to avoid bringing in fresh strains of the bacteria, and it should be noted specifically that acute greasy pig disease has been a common occurrence in repopulating herds following partial (feeding herd) depopulation (*see* Chapter 7). Where long-term problems with serious disease are seen, routine medication with in-feed antibiotics may be relevant. As an even longer term measure, autogenous vaccines can be produced under licence and injected back into pigs, either as a one- or two-dose programme. However, strain shift seems to occur and so such programmes have a limited lifespan until it is necessary to update the vaccine.

Oral Necrobacillosis or Facial Necrosis

This condition can be a manifestation of *Staphylococcus hyicus* infection, but it is far more common for *Fusiformes* spp. to be implicated. It results from skin infection of wounds, initially caused to the cheeks of baby piglets in the first forty-eight hours of life as a consequence of competition for teats. The eye-teeth (the corner incisor and canines) are present at birth as milk teeth and are needle-sharp (*see* Plate 12). In severe cases, piglets may be weakened by these severe lesions and suckling behaviour may be compromised, leading to death by starvation or overlaying.

Treatment
Nursing and assisted suckling will help young pigs with this condition, as will gentle bathing of lesions in 5 per cent soap solution.

Prevention
The condition can easily and readily be prevented by clipping or grinding all of the eight eye-teeth within twenty-four hours of birth, and in many pig-producing areas such a practice is routine. In other countries, its performance may be restricted (as in the UK) or completely banned (as in Norway).

Erysipelas

Disease caused by the ubiquitous bacteria *Erysipelothrix rhusiopathiae* (sometimes still called *Erysipelas insidiosa*) is common in pigs owing to their high susceptibility to infection. Erysipelas can cause reproductive failure in sows (*see* Chapter 1), but in the growing pig it produces lameness (*see* Chapter 9) or a septicaemic disease (*see* Chapter 11). It is included in this section because of the most obvious and well-recognized clinical signs, in which raised, hot, erythematous lesions appear, usually across the back of the pig. With a little imagination, these lesions can be seen to be diamond-shaped, thus giving the disease its common name of 'diamonds' (*see* Plate 13). The pig is likely to be depressed and inappetant, and will have a very high temperature (in excess of 42°C/108°F is common). Without treatment, death is likely. Sequelae to primary infection can occur, producing chronic lameness (*see* Chapter 9), sudden death as a result of heart lesions (endocarditis; *see* Chapter 11), and skin necrosis and sloughing (*see* Fig. 106).

Treatment and Control
If spotted and diagnosed early, treatment with penicillin is highly effective; temperatures will fall to normal within twelve hours, although a three-day course is often necessary to prevent chronic problems. In herd outbreaks, mass medication via water or feed – again with penicillin – is appropriate (note that despite *in vitro* studies, which suggest tetracyclines are

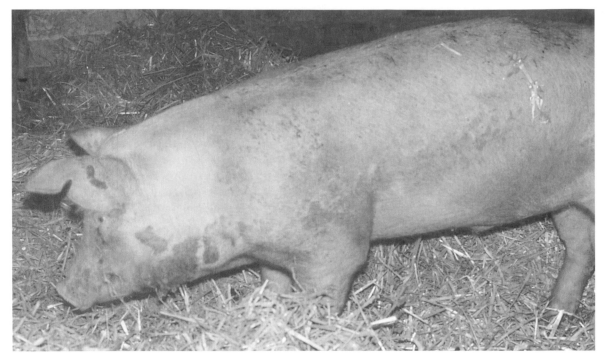

Fig. 106 Sloughing of the skin following necrosis in the advanced stage of, or recovery from, erysipelas.

effective at treating *Erysipelas rhusiopathiae*, this is not borne out in practice). In ideal conditions (for example, in deep straw bedding or in soil) the organism can persist for six months. As both wild birds and rodents are frequent asymptomatic carriers of the bacteria, control of disease must therefore involve the exclusion of both of these groups from pig-keeping pens and feed sources.

Prevention
Owing to the high susceptibility of the pig to erysipelas, vaccination of a breeding herd should be a standard policy. The bacteria is a weak antigen and, following a primary course of two doses, boosters are vital every six months. Commercial vaccines available usually cover serotypes 1 and 2 – the most common and generally held to be the most pathogenic – but if other serotypes are implicated, then autogenous vaccines are necessary. It should also be noted that erysipelas can become a long-term escalating problem in a breeding

herd, despite vaccination, where routine feedback (as described in Chapter 6) is performed. In such cases, feedback should cease.

In the growing herd, vaccination is not routine but can be used where necessary, usually as a single dose given at six to twelve weeks of age. However, long-term problems in growers can usually be prevented by attention to hygiene and exclusion of rodents and birds.

Other Bacterial Diseases
Following penetration of the integument, any environmental contaminant can produce lesions in or under the skin. Contamination of needles prior to, or during, injection is a common cause of subcutaneous abscesses that may be associated with *E. coli*, staphylococcal or streptococcal infection (*see* Fig. 107). Attention to hygiene of injection technique will therefore prevent such problems. However, infected abscesses of this sort should be differentiated from dry (in other words, sterile) abscesses that occur in response to mineral oil-

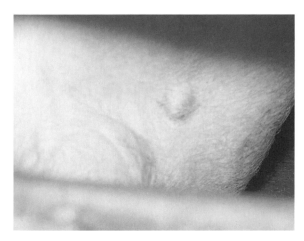

Fig. 107 A small abscess on the neck of a sow resulting from dirty injection technique.

based vaccines to which the pig reacts as if they are a foreign body. Such vaccines should be used only in breeding animals (to avoid carcass damage in slaughter pigs) and great operator care is needed as they can cause severe problems if accidentally self-injected. Other, more specific, agents that can rarely be implicated in skin lesions of the pig include the following.

Clostridia

Clostridium septicum and *C. chauvoei* are faeces- and soil-borne spore-forming bacteria that grow only in the absence of oxygen. Penetration of the skin accompanied by bruising can allow their colonization, and the powerful toxins they produce will lead to gas gangrene and rapid skin necrosis. Treatment with penicillin – if given early enough – will halt the multiplication and toxin production, although death may still occur in the early stages of the disease.

Spirochaetal Granuloma

Ulceration of the skin can lead to secondary infection with environmental spirochetes, producing a blackened weeping sore that, in the absence of treatment (antibiotics), will persist but remain localized. Such infection may be more common than is often diagnosed, as the primary ulcer (for example, on the shoulder or hock) forms the major concern and

laboratory tests on the secondary sore are rarely carried out.

Other Septicaemias
Any bacterium that becomes septicaemic will produce superficial or skin signs as part of the general disease. In particular, *Streptococcus suis*, *Haemophilus parasuis* and *Salmonella cholerae-suis* will all produce discoloration in the extremities (especially the ears, tail, vulva, lower limbs and teats) as circulation is compromised. These conditions are dealt with individually elsewhere.

VIRAL DISEASES

There are many viral diseases that affect the whole body of the pig, and these can present with skin signs. However, one virus that is implicated in a primary skin infection is pig pox.

Pig Pox

This is a rare disease that is difficult to confirm in samples and may occur congenitally (be present at birth). Historically, the spread of pig pox has been linked to lice and the rarity of this parasite may explain the low incidence of the disease. Typical pox lesions commence as reddened, round papules but rapidly develop a blackened centre, and they usually occur over the abdomen and between the back legs (*see* Plate 14). They may eventually form pustules, and secondary infection with *Staphylococcus hyicus* is common. Other than the congenital form affecting newborn pigs, mortality is rare and natural recovery tends to occur over a period of two to three weeks, providing secondary disease is controlled.

Treatment
There are no specific treatments.

Porcine Reproductive and Respiratory Syndrome (PRRS)

This major disease of pigs is covered in more detail in Chapters 1 and 7. However, it is included again here because in 1–2 per cent of cases skin lesions are produced, which will assist in

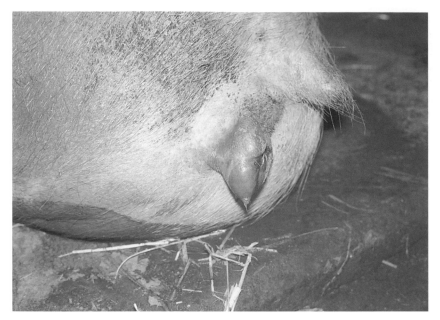

Fig. 108 Swollen and discoloured vulva associated with acute PRRS infection.

BELOW: *Fig. 109 Chemosis (swollen eyelids) in a neonatal piglet with PRRS.*

the diagnosis of an outbreak. Early colloquial terms for PRRS were 'blue ear disease' and 'abortus blauw', owing to the severe cyanosis affecting the ears (*see* Plate 15) and vulva (*see* Fig. 108) in acute and recovery phases of the infection. In addition, flushing of the skin may occur, particularly in sows (*see* Plate 16). In the newborn piglet infected prior to birth, the eyelids can be swollen (called chemosis; *see* Fig. 109) or the clotting mechanism may be compromised, rendering the pig very vulnerable to bruising following iron injection (*see* Plate 17).

Treatment and Control
The treatment and control of PRRS are dealt with in Chapters 1 and 7.

Porcine Dermatitis Nephropathy Syndrome (PDNS)

Included here as part of the post-weaning multisystemic wasting syndrome (*see* Chapters 6 and 7), PDNS is a recovery phase disease, probably as a result of a type III hypersensitivity reaction. It leads to occlusion of skin capillaries by antigen/antibody complexes, which in turn causes local necrosis and haemorrhage (*see* Plate 18). The kidneys are equally affected.

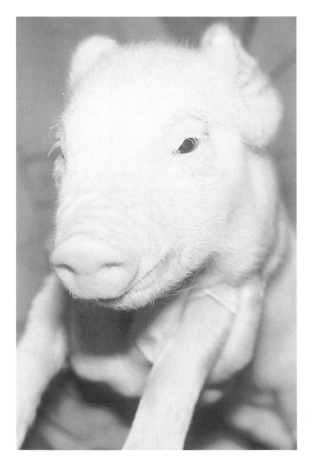

While outbreaks of this condition can occur in association with PMWS, it was first seen as a sporadic disease in Chile and the UK, mostly secondary to infection with other bacteria such as *E. coli*, *Actinobacillus pleuropneumoniae* and *Haemophilus parasuis*. *Pasteurella* has also been implicated, but porcine circovirus type II is now strongly linked with the condition.

Treatment
There is no treatment and farm experiences suggest mortality levels of 75 per cent are expected.

Prevention and Control
The prevention and control of PDNS rely upon identifying and managing the primary disease or trigger factors promoting PMWS in a herd.

Exotic Diseases
Some of the most devastating epizootic diseases of the pig can present with skin and surface lesions. Several of these diseases are of major worldwide importance, and are included on List A produced by the Office International des Épizooties (World Animal Health Organisation; *see* Chapter 13).

Vesicular Diseases
Of primary concern in this category are foot and mouth disease (FMD) and swine vesicular disease (SVD), but we should also include vesicular stomatitis (VS) and vesicular exanthena (VE). All produce primary vesicles on the snout and soft tissues of the foot (the coronary band and inter-digital space), and occasionally also on the teats, which ulcerate rapidly. FMD and SVD are clinically indistinguishable, but while FMD is a serious contagious disease (affecting all cloven-hoofed animals), SVD is mild and restricted to pigs. Owing to the difficulties of differentiation, however, many western countries have slaughter policies to cover both these diseases – as well as VS and VE – although in some areas vaccination is used to control disease. Vesicular exanthema is now seen only as a condition of sea mammals in California.

Swine Fevers
Both African and classical swine fever (hog cholera) are haemorrhagic diseases that can produce skin and other lesions grossly indistinguishable from PDNS. However, in most cases (although not necessarily all) the overall picture of disease – affecting all ages on a farm and producing persistent pyrexia – will enable differentiation from PDNS. Again, slaughter policies prevail in many of the world's major pig-producing areas such as the EU and North America.

PARASITIC DISEASES

Sarcoptic Mange
Sarcoptic mange is the result of infestation with *Sarcoptes scabei* var. *suis*, a mite that, while specific to the pig, is capable of producing mild disease in humans. It is physically indistinguishable from other subspecies of *Sarcoptes scabei* that are found in cats, rodents and humans, among others. The mite burrows into the skin to lay its eggs, which then slough off into the environment. There the eggs will mature to infective larvae to complete the life cycle, although they can also do so within the skin. The mites and eggs can survive outside the body (for a month or more in ideal conditions), which has important implications for both the perpetuation of disease within a population and eradication programmes.

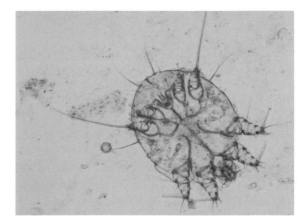

Fig. 110 The mange mite, Sarcoptes scabei *var.* suis.

Clinical Signs and Diagnosis
The single most significant sign of mange is pruritus, typically with rubbing, scratching, general unease and/or head shaking. In severe cases, condition loss can be significant, resulting in a knock-on effect to breeding efficiency in sows and a reluctancy in boars to work when encrusted. Growing pigs will incur lower feed efficiency when affected. Broadly, the disease can be split into three types:

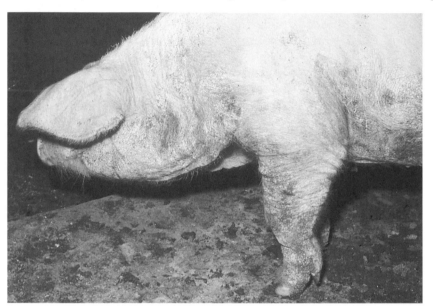

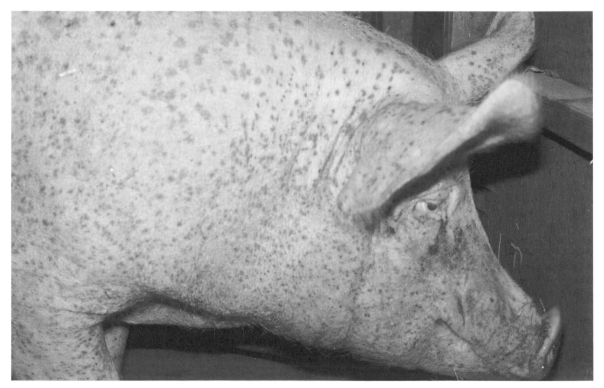

Fig. 111 Chronic encrusted mange, affecting wide areas of the body.

BELOW: *Fig. 112 Hypersensitivity to mange infestation.*

1. Acute infections following initial challenge (*see* Plate 19).
2. Chronic disease, mainly seen in adults and particularly affecting the ears, axillae and perineum.
3. Hypersensitivity, or allergic reaction.

Sarcoptic mange can usually be diagnosed clinically, and abattoir surveys can be used to access severity of herd disease. For confirmation, deep skin scrapings (particularly from the ears) will reveal mites, with the richest source of samples found in recently infected animals – in an enzootically infected herd these would be weaners weighing 20–30kg (45–65lb). Blood tests are also being developed as a diagnostic tool and may be used for health assurance purposes in seedstock.

Treatment
Ivermectins have revolutionized the treatment for mange, having now largely replaced organophosphorus-based products. They are given either parentally by injection or orally within the feed. The duration of treatment goes a long way to preventing reinfestation from the environment, although contact (direct or indirect) with other infected pigs will rapidly reinfect a treated animal.

Prevention and Control
The key to control of mange is based on breaking the cycle of infestation from pig to pig. Treatment of sows from two to seven days prior to moving into clean farrowing accommodation will allow a mange-free litter to be produced, and these will remain thus provided they do not come into contact with a contaminated environment or other infected pigs. Therefore, strict hygiene and all in/all out procedures are vital. Dynamic groups of sows and hospital pens are problem areas owing to permanent occupation and hence the maintenance of the mite's cycle. Boars are also often neglected from treatment programmes and are a rich source of mites. Whole-herd treatment programmes, combined with hygiene measures, have been developed to eliminate mange from farms, and careful selection and isolation of incoming stock will maintain this freedom. Transport vehicles can, however, be a common source of reinfestation.

Lice
Haematopinus suis is a blood-sucking louse that is now rarely seen in commercial pig herds, although it is more likely to occur in backyard pigs. In severe cases, irritation can be intense and may produce similar overall effects to mange (weight loss, reduced fertility and so on).

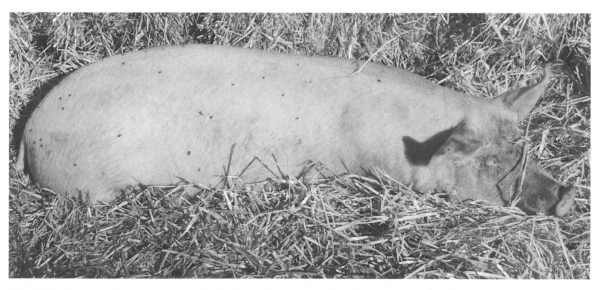

Fig. 113 The small black dots on the body of this pig are lice (Haematopinus suis).

The louse has a life cycle of around three to five weeks, which occurs wholly on the pig – the insect is able to survive only a matter of a few days off the body. Nits (lice eggs) are laid on the hairs.

Control
Lice are particularly significant as spreaders of disease within a population – any viraemic disease such as PRRS or swine fever will be spread by them, as will pig pox and eperythrozoonosis (*see* below). Therefore, control of lice is an integral part of the control of these diseases.

Other Insects
Biting flies and mosquitoes can be relevant in various parts of the world, with the latter in particular acting as a major vector of other diseases such as Japanese B encephalitis. Small papular lesions of sudden onset will be seen, although little adverse effect is noticed on the pig (*see* Plate 20). In warmer climates, soft ticks (*Ornithodoros* spp.) act as a long-term reservoir of infection for African swine fever, their bites spreading the virus from pig to pig. In heavy infestations, ticks may be seen attached to the pig primarily on the soft skin of the ventral abdomen and axillae.

Eperythrozoon suis
This is a blood-borne parasite that adheres to the surface of red blood cells and leads to their rupture, producing a haemolytic anaemia. Infection appears to be very widespread, but the role of this rickettsial agent in disease is somewhat unclear. In severe cases – possibly associated with the immunosuppressive effects of concurrent disease – condition loss, pallor and jaundice are the principal signs. The disease is debilitating and will have a significant effect on sow productivity if severe. Spread is by any means that transfers blood from pig to pig, including lice, biting flies, cannibalism and iatrogenic spread by multiple use of needles for injection. Diagnosis is based on clinical signs confirmed by direct-impression blood smears (serological tests are being developed).

Treatment
Treatment for fourteen days with tetracyclines will eliminate the organism from the pig, and widespread use of these antibiotics for other purposes in worldwide commercial pig production may have an incidental benefit in reducing *E. suis* infection.

Fungal Disease
Ringworm is a generally mild but widespread sporadic skin disease of pigs, and can be quite variable in presentation. The pig-specific ringworm *Microsporum nanum* will produce classic circular ringworm lesions (which should be distinguished from pityriasis rosea – *see* below), but this species has specific geographical distribution (it is, for example, present in Australia but absent from the UK). Cross-infection with other animal ringworm species is common, particularly with *Trichophyton mentagrophytes*, the rodent ringworm that can contaminate bedding materials, especially straw. Disease is especially widespread in outdoor sows, but the lesions are often seen as no more than 'dirty marks' and there is little irritation (*see* Plate 21). Contact with farm cats has led to ringworm infection with *M. canis*, particularly in young piglets as cats tend to frequent creep areas.

Treatment
Specific anti-fungal washes such as those based on enilcanozole are available, although they may not be licensed for pig use. In most cases, treatment is not worthwhile and self-cure will occur, although this can take some weeks.

NON-INFECTIOUS SKIN DISEASES

Pityriasis Rosea
Otherwise known as false ringworm, this is a sporadic inherited condition, starting in pigs four to six weeks of age and resolving itself within twenty weeks. Although it does look dramatic, it is of no clinical significance unless secondary infection (for example, with *Staphylococcus hyicus*) occurs. Rings commence on the ventral

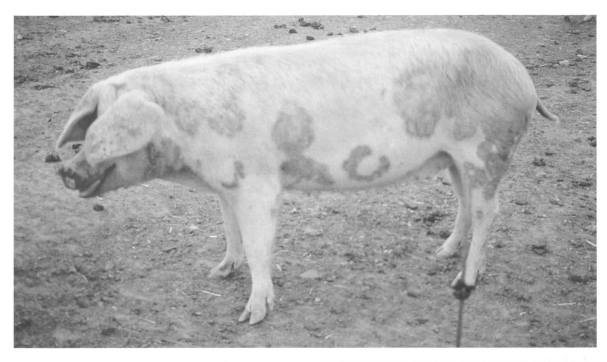

ABOVE: *Fig. 114 Ringworm in an outdoor sow, showing ring formation (contrast this with Plate 21, which is the more common manifestation of the condition).*

Fig. 115 Hyperkeratosis, or excessively flaky skin.

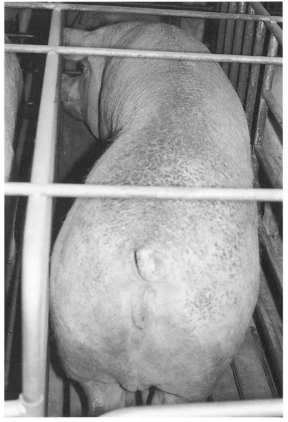

abdomen, enlarge, spread and coalesce to affect the whole body (*see* Plate 22). It is non-irritant.

Hyperkeratosis
Thickening, flaking and sloughing of the skin is often seen in adult pigs and must be differentiated from chronic mange. It is usually non-irritant, and the back, face and legs tend to be affected. The condition is most commonly seen in sows kept in stalls (especially under the water tank), but is of no health significance. Some breed types, such as Vietnamese Pot-Bellied Pigs, are particularly prone to hyperkeratosis.

Treatment and Prevention
If desired, the flaking skin can be removed by light scrubbing with a brush and 5 per cent soap solution, or by low-pressure power-washing

(less than 3.45bar/50psi is essential). Prevention can be effected by weekly application of light mineral oil produced for the purpose.

Epitheliogenesis Imperfecta

A congenital condition, thought to be inherited, in which the skin is not fully formed but is present in patches over the back or front of the 'knees' (*see* Fig. 116). In the latter case, it must be differentiated from knee abrasion (*see* below).

Treatment

Mildly affected animals will heal over time by scarring (provided there is no secondary infection), but severely affected animals should be destroyed. It is possible to use tape, sticking plaster or glue to protect affected knees as they heal.

Thrombocytopaenic Purpura

Primarily seen in pigs around ten to fourteen days of age, thrombocytopaenic purpura is a haemorrhagic disease resulting from the destruction of platelets by maternally derived antibodies, similar to the problems faced by human rhesus babies. A proportion of a litter is likely to be affected, and pigs are often

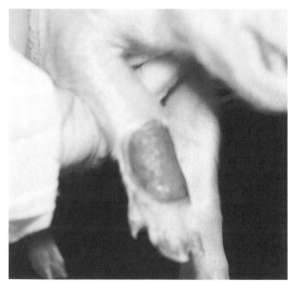

Fig. 116 Epitheliogenesis imperfecta. Lesions may also occur across the back.

found dead with small haemorrhages evident in the skin, particularly of the abdomen (*see* Plate 25). Haemorrhage is also widespread within the internal organs.

Treatment and Prevention

There is no treatment, but the disease must be differentiated from other haemorrhagic conditions such as the swine fevers and acute septicaemias (for example, that caused by *Actinobacillus suis*). Altering future breeding programmes will prevent subsequent litters being affected.

Dermatosis Vegetans

A rare condition causing congenital encrustation of the skin, particularly the legs, and accompanied by a fatal giant cell pneumonia, which develops over a period of two to three weeks.

Treatment and Prevention

This is another inherited condition and so treatment is neither effective nor appropriate. Instead, breeding programmes should aim to eliminate it from the herd.

SKIN DAMAGE AND INJURIES

Damage to the outer integument of the pig can broadly be split into two distinct groups:

1. That caused by interaction with the environment.
2. That caused by other pigs.

Environmental Damage

Any hard or sharp object can cause damage to the skin, but interaction with flooring probably accounts for most injuries of this nature in indoor commercial pig production. There are a number of distinct conditions that require consideration.

Sunburn

Of obvious cause and thus restricted to pigs exposed to open sunlight, sunburn (*see* Plate 24) is particularly seen in the early summer (May and June in Europe). When severe, it can prompt the pig to dip its back and walk on its 'knees', and blistering can be seen. In breeding gilts, reproductive failure (return to oestrus or abortion) is a common sequel to sunburn. Emollient cream can be used in severe cases to ease the discomfort.

Scald

Burning of the skin can result from contact with uncured limewash (*see* Plate 23), disinfectants or urine (transit erythema). Tethered sows on solid floors are particularly prone to urine scald around the perineum. Damage must be differentiated from acute ulcerative greasy pig disease (*see* page 115) and vesicular diseases (*see* page 123). If scalding occurs during transit, it can have serious implications for carcass or skin condemnation at slaughter.

Teat Necrosis

This is seen within the first few days of life and is of significance in that teats can be damaged to the extent that future milking ability is compromised in the breeding animal. Oestrogen levels rise during the parturition process and this leads to a hardening of the teats as they become engorged with blood. If the piglets are kept on bare concrete or rough floors, the front two or three pairs of their teats become damaged due to abrasion as they lie down to suck (*see* Plate 26).

Damage to teats can be prevented by the use of deep bedding, if appropriate, or by protecting the teats at birth with sticking plaster or insulation tape (although this must be removed after five days to prevent it cutting in). Alternatively, the teats can be painted with a skin-safe glue and then the pig dipped in a bowl of wood shavings; this forms a protective crust over the teats, which will gradually wear off over a few days.

Scuffed Knees

Again, this is the result of abrasion on the floor as the pig scrabbles to compete for a teat, although it must be differentiated from epitheliogenesis imperfecta (*see* page 128). Ulceration

of the skin can be so great that it penetrates the carpal (knee) joint, leading to septic arthritis (*see* Fig. 92).

Attention to rough floors and provision of deep bedding material, particularly in the first two days of life, will reduce damage. Suitable materials to use are chopped straw, shavings and shredded paper.

Ulcerative Bursitis

In older pigs, adventitious bursae can develop over pressure points. These are fluid-filled sterile cushions under the skin that result from continuous insult to any bony projections. The classic site is below and behind the hock (*see* Fig. 117). If flooring is of a poor standard, ulceration of the skin over this swelling occurs and granuloma formation results (*see* Plate 27). This may require surgical removal or culling of the pig on humane grounds.

The development of the initial bursitis is so widespread in indoor pigs as to be virtually ubiquitous. It is particularly a risk in pigs reared in deep-straw systems (as in outdoor pens) and then moved onto concrete floors. The ulceration is the result of abrasions with poor-quality floors, so attention to these will prevent problems.

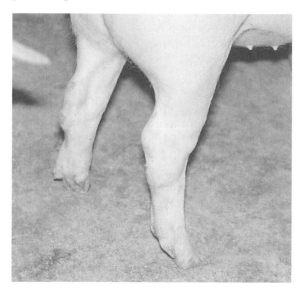

Fig. 117 A fluid-filled swelling below the hock, known as adventitious bursitis.

Shoulder Sores

These are seen almost exclusively in the breeding sow and are the result of skin ulceration over the point of the shoulder. The damage is the result of an interaction between the following factors:

1. The genetic (phenotypic) make-up of the sow – some sows have very prominent and protruding bone at the joint of the shoulder.
2. Excessive weight loss during lactation, removing the protective fat cushion over the shoulder.
3. Abrasion on farrowing-house floors. This is commonly seen in part-slatted houses where the back (slatted) area is slippery, making it difficult for the sow to rise. Oversized sows in restrictive crates are also at risk.

Once shoulder sores are present, the sow must be removed to a deep-straw area and, if the ulcer is deep, antibiotic treatment is appropriate. Carpet patches can also be glued over the ulcer to act as a protective pad. There is a tendency for the underlying bone to be damaged, leading to bony proliferation at the point of the shoulder, which is permanent. This renders the sow even more prone to future abrasion and ulceration. Prevention of shoulder sores depends upon attention to flooring and correct feed management of the breeding and lactating sow over her lifetime.

Damage Caused by Other Pigs

Damage from fighting has already been discussed with respect to the development of greasy pig disease and facial necrosis (*see* pages 115 and 119). We now turn to what can best be described as cannibalistic behaviour but which is often referred to as vice.

Growing Pigs

For the purposes of this summary, the various manifestations of vice in the growing pig will be considered together. These may occur as tail-biting, ear-biting (affecting the base of the ears, not the tips as in ear-tip necrosis) and flank- and stifle-biting. All have common origins.

Aberrant behaviour evidenced as vice is an extremely complex issue that involves interaction between environmental conditions, social conditions, nutrition and feed availability, genetics and health. Extremely long lists can be constructed of the factors that have been implicated, but for practical purposes the most significant of these are as follows:

1. Overstocking.
2. Draughts.
3. Inadequate feed availability.
4. Lack of opportunity to chew.
5. Concurrent serious health problems.

Control lies in identifying and correcting the underlying causes, but specific active measures to reduce aggression and vice include:

1. Tail docking early in life.
2. Raised salt levels in diets – up to 1 per cent sodium chloride can be added, so long as water is freely available.
3. Provision of chewable objects, preferably hanging in the pen. Chains and alkathene piping are suitable for this purpose.
4. Use of suitable bedding material. It is often claimed that provision of straw prevents tail-biting; this is not true, although it may help in some circumstances. Peat or used mushroom compost has been shown to be preferable to pigs, but this carries dangers associated with contamination (avian tuberculosis and salmonellae, respectively).
5. Early removal of a specific culprit.

Tail-biting is the most serious of the conditions as it can lead to secondary abscessation and paralysis, or be so severe as to require euthanasia on humane grounds.

Sows

Vulva-biting is a particular problem in loose-housed sows and tends to occur in late pregnancy. It is likely to be more common in dynamic groups but can be a major problem in specific fixed groups where there is one major culprit. The underlying cause appears to be

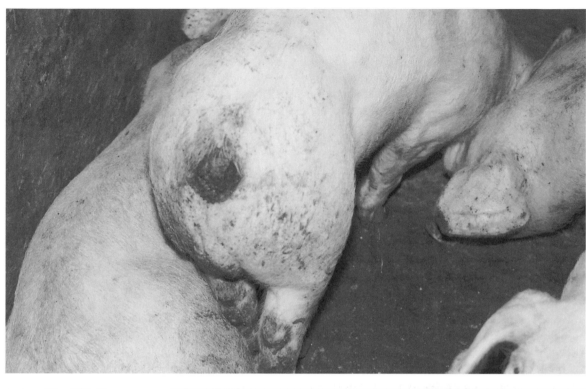

ABOVE: *Fig. 118 Severe tail-bite lesions.*

Fig. 119 Damage over the stifle area – biting or floor abrasion?

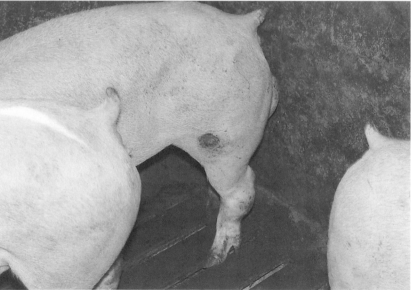

associated with feed intake involving low-volume high-specification diets. Use of bulk feed, such as sugar-beet pulp or potato waste, will prevent aggression, and generally less vulva-biting is seen in sows housed on barley straw compared to wheat, rape, pea or oat straw.

The design of the races in electronic sow feeders – particularly older types with rear exit gates – may be associated with a different set of problems. Damage caused by such systems can be so great as to cause obstruction to the farrowing process or even subsequent service. In such sows culling is necessary, although if they do become pregnant emergency episiotomy may be needed at farrowing where scarring obstructs the birth canal.

Superficial Swellings
A range of conditions can produce swelling, either under or within the skin, which will be obvious to the observer. Such swelling can be the result of injury, developmental abnormality or infection.

Bruises and Abscesses
Physical damage by other pigs or as a result of contact with hard structures can lead to the rupture of blood vessels under the skin and consequent leakage of blood, in some cases producing huge swellings. If these are inconvenient to the pig they can be surgically drained, but great care is needed to avoid contamination and subsequent abscessation.

Abscesses may also occur as a result of penetration of the skin, either through fighting or, specifically, following poor injecting technique. Drainage and subsequent flushing of the abscess with clean water should precede antibiotic therapy.

Ear Lesions
Haematomas in the ear are specific blood blisters, resulting from rupture of deep ear veins (*see* Fig. 120). They can be caused by fighting or by contact with equipment such as feed hoppers, but most significantly they are seen as a result of head shaking in association with sarcoptic mange (*see* page 123). These lesions should be drained surgically only if the pig is severely compromised; otherwise, they should be left alone, in which case the blood will be reabsorbed to leave a 'cauliflower ear' (*see* Fig. 121).

Swelling as a result of infection from ear tags is a common problem, particularly in sows. When this is seen, the tag should be removed, the swelling drained and antibiotics administered.

HERNIAS AND RUPTURES

Two major types of hernias are seen in the pigs: inguinal hernias and umbilical hernias.

Inguinal Hernia, or Ball Rupture
Here, the inguinal ring in the groin is enlarged, causing intestinal loops and fat to pass through and become evident in the scrotum (*see* Fig. 122). The lesions are the result of an inherited defect in the inguinal ring. Affected pigs can still be castrated but only by a closed technique.

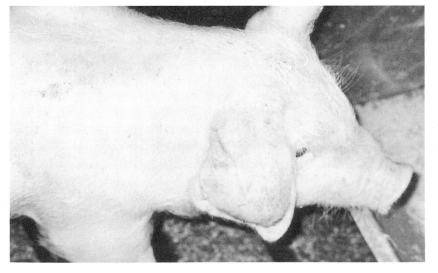

Fig. 120 Swelling of the ear as a result of aural haematomas.

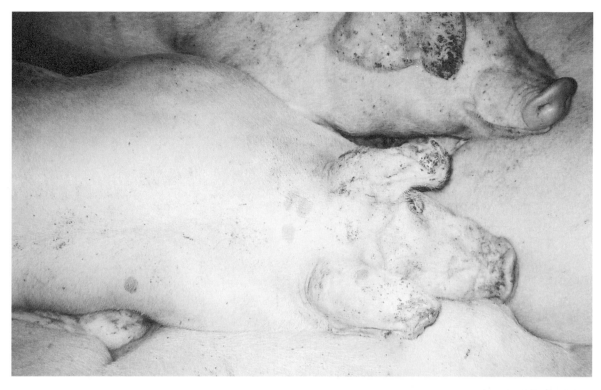

Fig. 121 Cauliflower ear following reabsorption of the haemotoma.

Fig. 122 Massive inguinal hernia.

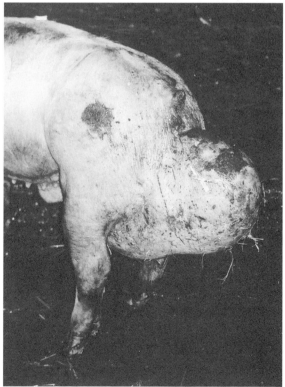

Uncastrated pigs can still grow to slaughter weight, although the hernias in some may become so large as to require humane destruction of the boar. Rarely, the gut loops will become entrapped and the pig will rapidly die with wet gangrene. (Inguinal hernias can occur in gilts but are rare. In such cases the swelling will be seen in the groin area and stretch down over the front of the stifle joint.)

Umbilical Hernia, or Ruptures

Here, the hole in the abdominal wall through which the umbilical cord passed in the foetus becomes enlarged and, again, gut loops pass through (*see* Fig. 123). These hernias can become very large and abraded, such that euthanasia is required, but small areas can still permit growth to slaughter. Surgical repair is not economically viable.

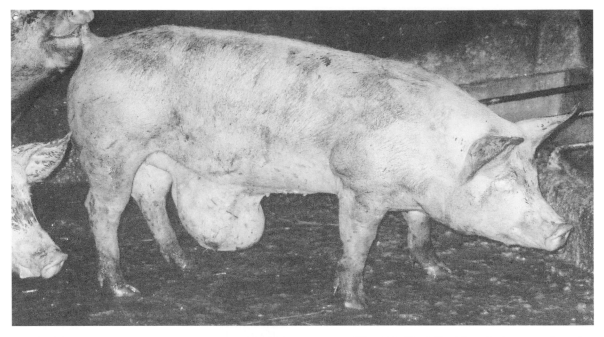

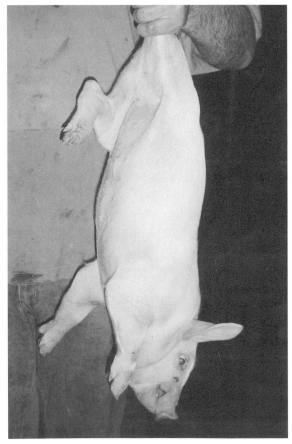

ABOVE: *Fig. 123 Umbilical hernia in a growing pig.*

Fig. 124 Lifting a young pig by one back leg creates sheering forces on the longitudinal abdominal muscles and can trigger umbilical herniation.

The causes of umbilical hernia are complex. There may be an inherited weakness in the abdominal wall that is exacerbated by infection in the navel (the result of sucking by other pigs), especially after weaning and handling. In addition, lifting a heavy pig by one back leg will create a shearing force on the abdominal musculature, such that the umbilicus opens up to allow herniation. Pigs should therefore always be lifted by two legs.

The nature and colour of the skin of the pig, particularly the predominantly white breeds, render it quite easy to see and distinguish lesions. The pig is susceptible to a wide range of skin diseases and abnormalities, as well as superficial swellings, many of which can be diagnosed accurately by the experienced eye. However, laboratory testing still has a confirmatory role in many instances.

CHAPTER ELEVEN

Septicaemia and Sudden Death

SEPTICAEMIA

A range of bacterial infections can gain entry to the body and spread via the bloodstream to all organs to produce the pathological signs of septicaemia. Figure 125 lists the common bacteria found, along with the age groups of pigs most likely to be affected by them. Most of these conditions have been covered in previous chapters; those that have not are discussed below.

The features of any septicaemia are similar, both clinically and at post-mortem examination, and the various causes can be differentiated only by laboratory examination. However, in an outbreak of disease within a population, other signs of the infection may be seen in less severely affected individuals (for example, 'diamonds' in cases of erysipelas).

Septicaemia presents as a very acute onset illness, in which some pigs may simply be found dead. If still alive, they will have a pyrexia (often up to 42°C/108°F) and be severely depressed. They are unlikely to be eating or drinking, usually just lie around and are reluctant to rise, and respiratory rates will be increased. There is often discoloration of the skin, particularly of the extremities, with anything from red to black areas forming in the ears, tail, lower limbs and genitals. In rare recovered cases, sloughing of dead skin from these areas may be seen. There will also often be hyperaemia (increased blood flow) to the skin of the abdomen and ventral chest (*see* Plate 28). Death usually occurs within a few hours, the animal entering a comatose state prior to this happening.

Fig. 125 Bacteria causing septicaemia and the age groups most at risk from each.

Organism	Age group most at risk
Actinobacillus suis	Sucking piglets
Salmonella cholerae-suis	Weaners and growers
Streptococcus suis	Sucking piglets/weaners
Haemophilus parasuis	Weaners to adults
Erysipelothrix rhusiopathiae (erysipelas)	Growers to adults
Escherichia coli	Sucking piglets and weaners
Bacillus anthracis (anthrax)	Weaners and young growers
Leptospira (*L. canicola* or *L. icterohaemorrhagiae*)	Sucking piglets

At post-mortem examination, changes will be noted in most major systems. There will be minute haemorrhages on swollen kidneys, liver, lungs, heart, spleen and intestinal wall, and excessive fluid may be present in the chest, pericardium and abdomen. Rigor mortis may not occur in animals that have died with a high temperature and clotting of the blood may be delayed. Bacteriological sampling of heart blood and affected tissues from an untreated animal will yield a pure growth of the causative organisms.

Specific Agents of Septicaemia

Aside from septicaemia-causing bacteria discussed in previous chapters, infection by the following agents can also lead to the disease.

Actinobacillus suis

This bacterium is commonly found in pig populations and rarely causes disease. Where septicaemia does occur, it is normally found in young piglets and the whole litter may be affected. It does not appear to spread from litter to litter, suggesting that it may be related to deficiencies in either colostrum quality or intake. The pigs are normally found dead and may show some ventral skin haemorrhages reminiscent of thrombocytopaenic purpura (*see* page 128). Treatment of unaffected littermates or very early cases with a broad-spectrum synthetic penicillin such as amoxycillin can be successful.

It should be noted here that *Actinobacillus suis* has occasionally been seen as a cause of skin vesicular disease – to be differentiated from foot and mouth disease and swine vesicular disease (*see* page 123). It may also cause discreet lung lesions in slaughter pigs, which are indistinguishable from chronic *Actinobacillus pleuropneumoniae* lesions.

Salmonella cholerae-suis

This species of *Salmonella* is unique in that it produces a septicaemic disease in pigs, in contrast with the usual enteric infection in most other species. There is a strong association between the incidence of *Salmonella cholerae-suis* and classical swine fever, and its occurrence in western Europe reflects the disappearance of the latter.

This species of *Salmonella* is pig-specific and is spread by the movement of, usually, weaner pigs and their effluent. It is not zoonotic. Control of rare outbreaks of disease will depend on accurate diagnosis and selection of antimicrobials based on sensitivity testing. In intractable situations, autogenous vaccines may be produced, and in some countries commercial vaccines are available.

Bacillus anthracis (Anthrax)

The bacterial infection anthrax is notifiable in many countries and leads to an acute septicaemia in growing pigs, with a tendency to produce oedema in the neck. While the disease is highly sensitive to penicillin, the risks to both humans and other animal species – particularly through the ability of *Bacillus anthracis* to sporulate, producing spores that can survive and remain infective for many years – means that state control is most likely. In particular, control of the spread of manure or slurry from an infected farm must be tightly restricted to prevent the spread of disease.

Leptospirosa

The role of *Leptospira bratislava* is discussed in Chapter 1. However, many species of *Leptospira* are capable of inducing septicaemic disease in young piglets, in particular *L. canicola* (derived from dogs) and *L. icterohaemorrhagiae* (derived from rats). In addition to normal septicaemia signs, severe jaundice may be a feature of the carcass, resulting from either renal or hepatic damage.

These forms of leptospirosis are very rare, despite the close proximity of pigs and rats in many farms. Prevention rests with maintaining separation of pigs from the source species and their waste (particularly urine). Early treatment with streptomycin is effective, provided the damage done is not too advanced. While vaccines against these two species of bacteria are commonly used in dogs, this is not the case in pigs.

Other Acute Pyrexic Diseases

Sudden-onset high fever and rapid death can be a feature of a wide range of viral diseases in addition to the bacterial septicaemias discussed above. Examples include classical swine fever (hog cholera), African swine fever, foot and mouth disease, Nipah virus, Teschan virus and Aujeszky's disease. All are controlled in most major pig-producing regions by state programmes, but they must be borne in mind in the event of sudden deaths, particularly those associated with fever, and in cases where deaths occur simultaneously in a wide range of ages.

SUDDEN DEATH

It should be noted here that 'sudden death' and 'found dead' are not necessarily the same thing. Animals that are found dead in a modern commercial farm situation may quite easily have developed an illness over a few hours without being seen and then died. This is very different to the case of a perfectly normal animal that dies within minutes. However, for practical purposes the two groups must be linked together, and differentiation of the wide range of causes can be made only at post-mortem examination. A list of these causes and the age of pig affected is given in Figure 126; septicaemia and exotic viral disease, discussed above, must also be included here.

Precipitating Earlier Disease and Damage

A number of animals that have been exposed to specific diseases and have either recovered or have not shown signs of the disease may be found dead weeks or months after the primary infection. Three main causes are responsible for this: endocarditis, pericarditis and strangulation of hernias.

Endocarditis

This condition involves the growth of colonies of bacteria on the heart valves secondary to bacteraemic spread. The most common bacteria implicated include *Erysipelothrix rhusiopathiae*, *Streptococcus suis* type II, *Actinobacillus suis* and *E. coli*, although any other circulating bacteria could be involved. When the lesions reach a certain size, circulatory collapse occurs and the pig may literally drop dead. Prevention of such lesions depends on diagnosis of the bacteria involved and control programmes designed to attend to the primary disease condition.

Pericarditis

Pericarditis is an inflammation of the sac containing the heart as a result of septicaemic disease earlier in life, such that this sac forms a constriction around the heart. As the pig grows (and hence the heart grows with it) the constriction gets tighter, until eventually the heart will fail – often following some physical activity such as moving and mixing. Pericarditis lesions can also commonly be found at slaughter, having apparently caused no significant effect on the pig's growth or health.

Severe chronic pericarditis is believed to be a result of challenge from one of three agents: *Haemophilus parasuis*, *Streptococcus suis* and *Mycoplasma hyorhinis*. As with endocarditis, the prevention of sudden deaths from pericarditis rests with control of the primary disease.

Hernia Strangulation

Strangulation of a long-standing umbilical or inguinal hernia (*see* pages 132–4) can occur at any time. The effect is the same as with a twisted gut (*see* pages 66–7), in that there is obstruction to the blood supply, leading to gangrenous changes to the gut and releasing powerful endotoxins that cause death by endotoxic shock. Death as a result of strangulation of hernias will occur two to six hours after the event.

Primary Heart Failure

Congenital abnormalities of the heart exist in some pigs, and such animals will usually either die or be euthanized before weaning. The various types of defect described in other species (such as hole in the heart and persistent

Cause	Common age affected
Septicaemias	Baby piglets to adults
Acute viral disease	Baby piglets to adults
Endocarditis	Growers and adults
Pericarditis	Growers
Porcine dermatitis nephropathy syndrome	Growers
Strangulation of hernias	Growers
Torsion of intestine	Growers and sows
Gastric dilation and torsion	Adults
Fighting injury	Growers and adults
Primary heart failure	Piglets and adults
Porcine stress syndrome	Growers and adults
Mulberry heart disease	Weaners and growers
Hepatosis dietetica	Weaners and growers
Phenol poisoning	Weaners and growers
Aflatoxin poisoning	Weaners and growers
Acute *Actinobacillus pleuropneumoniae* infection	Growers
Gastric ulceration	Growers and adults
Porcine haemorrhagic enteropathy	Growers and adults
Clostridium novyi infection	Growers and adults
Heatstroke	Growers and adults
Salt poisoning	Growers
Cystitis/pyelonephritis	Adult sows
Electrocution	Any age
Asphyxiation and suffocation	Any age
Fire	Any age

Fig. 126 Ages commonly associated with selected causes of sudden death.

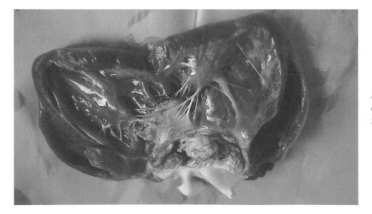

Fig. 127 Cauliflower lesions developing on the heart valves, typical of endocarditis.

ductus arteriosus) are poorly described in the pig. Of far greater significance is primary heart failure in sows, often occurring around the time of farrowing.

The heart of the pig has been described as having a number of peculiarities, such as low volume and small weight compared with total body size, abnormal blood volume capacities and high sensitivity of the heart muscle to oxygen deprivation. This means that whenever the heart is placed under increased demand – as takes place when moving, farrowing, fighting and so on – it has a tendency to go into myocardial failure. The larger the animal, the greater the risk – hence the level of problems seen in the sow. The sensitivity to lack of oxygen may also explain the sudden death of some pigs with extensive lung damage, which would not, in itself, be expected to be fatal.

A heart in which the muscle has failed will be flabby and surrounded by a small amount of pericardial fluid. Other signs of acute heart failure may be present at post-mortem, such as congestion or oedema of the lungs, pleural and peritoneal exudate, and congestion of blood in other major organs such as the liver and lungs.

Mulberry Heart Disease (MHD) and Hepatosis Dietetica (HD or Herztod)

As part of the normal metabolic function, waste products are broken down prior to excretion. A wide range of chemical processes are involved in this, one of which, if left unchecked, involves a damaging oxidation process that yields free radicals in the form of toxic peroxides. These free radicals are highly damaging to tissues, and to prevent their excess production in the body an antioxidant system exists. In the pig, by far and away the most important antioxidants are vitamin E (alpha-tocopherol) and selenium. Problems can arise with the antioxidant system in two specific circumstances: a shortage of either or both of these micronutrients; or an increased requirement for antioxidants.

Mulberry heart disease (MHD) and hepatosis dietetica (HD) both present in the same way –

sudden death – and are both a reflection of a shortage of antioxidants. There is a suggestion that MHD may be more than simply the manifestation of vitamin E deficiency, and HD is more likely to result from selenium deficiency. MHD is common in commercial pig-production systems, while HD is comparatively rare.

Diagnosis

The diagnosis of either condition is based upon the circumstances of the sudden death and typical post-mortem findings. MHD death will literally be sudden and is usually seen post-weaning up to eight to ten weeks of age in well-grown pigs, although in rare circumstances it can be seen pre-weaning. It is particularly a feature of fast-growing weaners. At post-mortem examination there may be congestion of the carcass and blood pooling under the skin. The heart will be surrounded either by fluid or jelly, and it will be covered in haemorrhagic flecks that penetrate throughout the heart muscle. The lungs will be oedematous (wet) and the interlobular septa will be very obvious. There may be small amounts of excess fluid in the abdomen and the liver will tend to be enlarged as a result of blood accumulation.

Hepatosis dietetica tends to occur in slightly older pigs three to four months of age but still presents as sudden death. The liver will be swollen and mottled, and it will frequently have ruptured, leading to haemorrhage into the abdomen. The consistency of the liver is crumbly compared to the normal pig's liver, which is firm and resilient.

Prevention

Selenium is normally included in pig rations at a rate of 3mg per kg and, in most cases, this will protect against deficiency and hence hepatosis dietetica. Selenium is, however, highly toxic, and so care is needed with supplementation.

Dosing with vitamin E to prevent MHD is far more complex. At birth, the pig has a reserve of vitamin E derived transplacentally and hence is dependent upon the vitamin E supply given to the sow during pregnancy. There is minimal

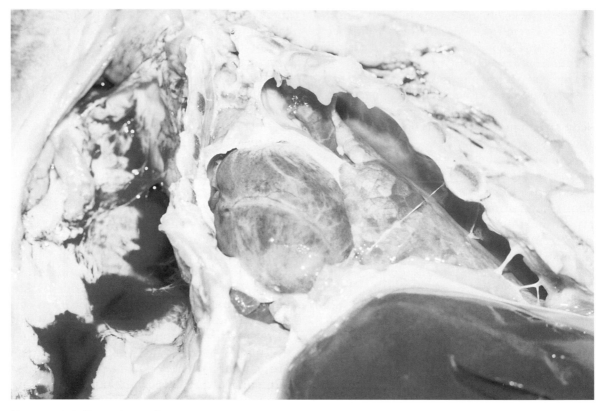

Fig. 128 Mulberry heart disease.

transfer of vitamin E via the milk and, thus, body levels decline during the sucking phase. The faster the pigs grow, the more rapidly these reserves will be used up. At weaning, blood levels of vitamin E drop even more rapidly and starter diets are required to provide the total needs. However, there appears to be a time lag of two to three weeks between dietary intake and beneficial effect on the body. Thus, if the pigs are born with inadequate levels of vitamin E and use up their reserves rapidly, they will become deficient in the immediate post-weaning period, irrespective of the dietary levels in the starter diet. MHD beyond two to three weeks post-weaning hence indicates a deficient starter diet, whereas earlier death suggests that the dry sow diet is deficient.

Where death from MHD occurs immediately or soon after weaning, the following prevention strategies are needed:

1. Injection of pigs at weaning with vitamin E/selenium supplement.
2. Water supplementation with soluble vitamin E – usually included in multivitamin preparation.
3. Water supplementation with vitamin C – an alternative and less essential antioxidant, but one that is both rapidly absorbed and protective.
4. In the longer term, dry sow dietary levels of vitamin E should be reviewed.

Where death occurs later, it is the post-weaning diets that require evaluation for vitamin E/selenium levels.

In addition to the high susceptibility of fast-growing young pigs to MHD, a number of other factors can precipitate it. These, however, can easily be addressed so that the condition is prevented from occurring in the herd:

1. Decay of vitamin E levels in storage – always observe the use by dates on feed.
2. Destruction of vitamin E by heat or acidity in storage.
3. High levels of polyunsaturated fatty acids (for example, soya oil) in diets, which increase the requirement for antioxidants.
4. The presence of the halothane gene in the carrier state (*see* below).

Commercial pig diets contain varying levels of vitamin E. A summary is given in Figure 129.

Diet	Vitamin E levels
Dry sow diets	60–100IU/kg
Lactation diets	60–100IU/kg
Creep and starter diets	150–200IU/kg
Weaner diets	100–150IU/kg
Grower/finisher diets	50–100IU/kg

Note: in slow-growing pigs (for example, for niche product yield) such high levels are not necessary, but nor are they harmful.

Fig. 129 Typical levels of vitamin E in commerical pig diets.

Porcine Stress Syndrome (PSS)

Otherwise known as malignant hyperthermia, porcine stress syndrome is a genetically based inherited condition caused by the presence of the so-called halothane gene. It is characterized by rapid death following an uncontrolled rise in body temperature, and is typically seen in weaners and growers, although susceptible sows are also sometimes affected. Death normally occurs following some minor or major stress such as moving, fighting or transportation, but in sows it can occur at farrowing and even at mating time.

The truly susceptible pig is homozygous positive for the halothane gene, having inherited one of these recessive genes from each of its parents. The name of the gene is derived from the fact that, up until the early 1990s, susceptible pigs were identified by their reaction to the anaesthetic gas halothane (they go into malignant hyperthermia, characterized by a rapidly rising tempertaure, muscular spasms and death). Nowadays, a DNA gene test, based on blood samples, can be used to detect both the homozygous susceptible pig (hh) and the carrier pig (Hh). (H is used to represent the normal gene, while h indicates the recessive halothane gene.)

Affected pigs will be usually found dead, will have a very rapid onset of rigor mortis and will be pale. The body temperature may also still be elevated when the animal is found. At post-mortem examination, the muscle will be pale with a 'part-cooked' appearance; this is most noticeable in the major muscle masses of the hind legs and in the longissimus dorsi (eye muscle). It is also a particular feature of heavily muscled pigs that have grown well (*see* Plate 29).

Fully stress-susceptible populations of pigs are generally restricted to specific breed types – in particular, the Pietrain and certain Landrace lines. However, the incorporation of these breed types into hybrids in the 1980s meant that the halothane gene became common within breeding and, hence, feeding pig populations. Moreover, it was found that the presence of the halothane gene (in carrier pigs, Hh) produced a benefit in terms of lean tissue deposition (muscle growth), and so a number of seedstock suppliers specifically produced terminal sires that carried the gene, passing it on to 50 per cent of their offspring to gain this benefit.

Later on in the 1980s, it became apparent that even carrier pigs were susceptible to a form of PSS. In populations using these carrier boars, mortality levels of 4 per cent in growers due to PSS were not uncommon. This incidence was too high to be accounted for by the low level of the halothane gene in the female population, which would produce a small number of homozygous (hh) offspring when mated to a carrier boar. Hence, some of the carriers (Hh) must also be susceptible in an as yet unknown way.

Halothane gene in parent and FI generation	Comments
Parents: HH × Hh Offspring: 50% HH, 50% Hh	Not stress susceptible, 50% carriers
Parents: HH × hh Offspring: 100% Hh	Not stress susceptible, 100% carriers
Parents: Hh × Hh Offspring: 25% HH, 50% Hh, 25% hh	25% stress susceptible, 50% carriers
Parents: Hh × hh Offspring: 50% Hh × 50% hh	50% stress susceptible, 50% carriers
Parents: hh × hh Offspring: 100% hh	100% stress susceptible
Parents: HH × HH Offspring: 100% HH	Stress-free, no carriers

H = normal gene (dominant);
h = halothane gene (recessive).

*Fig. 130
Inheritance of the
halothane gene.*

Prevention

High levels of vitamin E and the inclusion of other antioxidant preparations in diets has been found to have some protective effect, even though vitamin E deficiency and PSS are distinct and separate entities.

The presence of the halothane gene in the slaughter generation has been associated with the production of pale soft exudative (PSE) meat in the slaughterhouse. For this reason and the increased occurrence of sudden death, combined with the ability to screen out the halothane gene by blood testing, European and North American seedstock producers have largely attempted to eliminate the gene from their populations and so the incidence of PSS in pigs has fallen. In particular, the numbers of 'dead on arrival' pigs at the slaughterhouse has fallen dramatically. However, PSS remains a concern in specific nucleus populations, particularly those involving the Pietrain breed.

Phenol Poisoning

Phenols are acutely toxic to pigs, causing massive liver damage and rapid death. At postmortem, the liver is distinctive: it is enlarged and friable, and lobules are clearly demarcated (*see* Fig. 131). If the pig has survived for even a few hours, jaundice may be seen throughout the carcass. The condition is more likely to occur in weaner pigs, although all ages are susceptible. Potential sources of phenols for pigs are creosote-treated wood, tarmac floors, phenolic disinfectants, tar-based waterproof sealant and clay pigeons (these are bound together by tar).

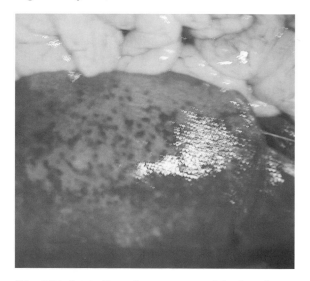

Fig. 131 Acute liver damage seen with phenol poisoning.

Episodes of phenol poisoning have been seen in outdoor-reared weaners over several months as kennels are moved across a field for sequential batches of pigs. As the kennels lie over an area in which clay pigeons have fallen, the young pigs consume them. If the problem is not diagnosed, it will disappear as subsequent batches are penned over 'clean' ground.

Prevention
Clearly, prevention of contact with any phenol-based product will ensure this problem does not occur.

Acute Mycotoxin Poisoning

Toxins produced by fungi (mycotoxins) can cause a wide range of effects in pigs, including reproductive problems (in the case of zearalenone – *see* page 20) and immune suppression (for example, with trichothecenes and ochratoxin A). Toxicity tends to be accumulative, with low levels of toxins taken in over a period time and limiting growth. However, occasionally acute aflatoxicosis is seen where dietary levels of aflatoxin exceed 2,000ppb; death in such cases may occur rapidly following a short period of depression. As with phenol poisoning, the liver is irreparably damaged and will be pale or tan-coloured, often with haemorrhagic flecks.

Mycotoxins are produced by fungi that infect feedstuffs, both during its growth and its storage. Mouldy straw may be a source, although levels are unlikely to reach those needed for acute toxicity to occur. Mould production within feed bins represents a high risk of mycotoxins.

Clostridium novyi (*oedematiens*) Infection

The clostridia group of bacteria produce powerful toxins that are involved in the putrefaction process after death. The organisms are present in the gut and their spores are found in soil. *Clostridium novyi* (type B) is a species that has the ability to track up from the intestine via the bile duct and enter the liver. Here, it proliferates rapidly, producing toxins that cause putrefaction and fermentation. The organism thrives in the absence of oxygen (hence its role in body decomposition after death), and it has been suggested that pigs with respiratory disease (where liver oxygen levels may be compromised) are more susceptible. However, in most cases examined post-mortem, there will be some evidence of inflammation in the intestine. This may facilitate bacterial proliferation in the gut and/or ascension of the bile duct, which connects to the upper reaches of the small intestine.

Post-mortem examination must be carried out immediately if a firm diagnosis is to be made, as liver decomposition will occur after death in an unaffected dead animal. The disease is usually seen in larger growing pigs and adults, which are found dead with a swollen discoloured abdomen. There will be a strong smell of decomposition; the liver will be swollen and dark bloody fluid will be present in the abdomen. On section, the liver will be full of gas bubbles, giving it the appearance of Aero chocolate (*see* Plate 30). Diagnosis can be confirmed by the demonstration of *Clostridium novyi* on impression smears of the cut surface of the liver by way of a fluorescent antibody test.

Prevention
Where a herd problem is identified, vaccination of sows using a multivalent clostridial vaccine is an effective preventative measure.

Heatstroke and Sunstroke

Compared to many mammals the pig is relatively poor at controlling its body temperature, a feature that tends to be exacerbated in the conditions in which pigs are kept. In particular, the pig lacks sweat glands and, thus, is limited in its methods of heat loss. Panting is the primary physiological mechanism for dissipating heat and, while blood flow to the ears can be increased to dissipate heat, this is relatively ineffective. The most effective method employed by the pig to lose heat is by wallowing and then allowing the latent heat of vaporization to cool the body.

Heatstroke is seen in two specific circumstances:

1. Outdoors in unprotected environments where no shade or wallows are provided, when adults are usually affected most. The incidence of heatstroke rises rapidly when environmental temperatures exceed 35°C (95°F), and the effects of direct sunshine are additive.
2. In heavily stocked, underventilated buildings when heat generation from the pigs outstrips the rate of hot-air removal from the building.

If seen alive, pigs will be in obvious respiratory distress (panting heavily), will be recumbent and will have a rectal temperature that may exceed 43°C (110°F). Many may simply be found dead. At post-mortem examination the body will be congested and, in particular, the lungs will be heavily congested. There may be variable amounts of bloody froth emanating from the nostrils. Diagnosis is normally based upon the clinical and post-mortem picture and through the elimination of other causes of death.

Treatment and Prevention

When seen alive, spraying with water and using tranquillizers to lower blood pressure may assist recovery. Prevention is based upon good husbandry, avoiding overstocking and underventilation, and providing shade and, in particular, wallows for outdoor sows that are otherwise unable to find shelter during hot weather. Restricting the amount of straw in arcs and using insulated/ventilated arcs will assist heat dissipation and reduce the air temperature inside, thereby lowering the chances of litter desertion.

Asphyxiation/Suffocation

Normal clean air contains 20.5 per cent oxygen and this is necessary for health. Expired air contains an increased percentage of carbon dioxide and a decreased percentage of oxygen, so it must be replenished with fresh air if pigs are to remain healthy. Furthermore, within the pigs' environment, other gases may be produced that are either directly poisonous themselves or have a competitive effect on the partial pressure of oxygen in the air. Asphyxiation is periodically seen in young and growing pigs in a range of circumstances, discussed below.

Lack of Oxygen

In power-ventilated buildings, a loss of power – either due to power failure or management error in not switching on fans after washing – will lead to a failure to replenish stale air. The oxygen partial pressure gradually will drop, eventually reaching the point where large numbers of pigs suffocate. This problem is seen particularly in winter when low ambient temperatures prevent high-temperature alarms from setting off (in warm weather situations, temperatures will rise to a level that sets off these alarms before the amount of oxygen is dangerously depleted). In such cases, whole rooms of pigs will be found dead, and no specific lesions are visible at post-mortem examination save for bloody froth around the nose and congested lungs.

The provision of fail-safe air inlets and outlets that are based upon loss of power rather than temperature, combined with adequate alarm systems, will prevent such disasters.

Carbon Monoxide Poisoning

When propane or butane gas is burnt, carbon dioxide and water vapour are produced. Where gas-powered heaters are used – either as creep lamps in farrowing areas or as heaters in weaning accommodation – adequate ventilation is therefore needed to remove these waste products. More seriously, however, are situations where heaters are badly maintained and burn inefficiently, such that carbon monoxide is produced. This gas competitively binds to haemoglobin in the blood, excluding oxygen and leading to anoxia and death. It is a heavy gas and drops to the floor, and so in the farrowing area death may be seen in young piglets without apparent problems in the sow (stillbirth is also a feature of carbon monoxide poisoning). In tiered weaning cages, the lower cages are also more likely to be affected.

Tissues and blood in pigs that have died of carbon monoxide poisoning are a bright cherry-red colour but no other specific signs are evident. Unexplained multiple deaths of young pigs in gas-heated accommodation should always raise the alert to carbon monoxide poisoning.

Hydrogen Sulphide Poisoning

Hydrogen sulphide is a highly toxic gas smelling of rotten eggs, which is given off from slurry stored under pigs. It can be released in farm slurry when agitated and, as a heavy gas, tends to hang close to the floor rather than being removed by upper-level fans. The highest risks arise when slurry is released from pits while the building is occupied. The sudden death of large numbers of pigs within a room following removal of slurry should therefore raise the possibility of hydrogen sulphide poisoning. This gas is also highly toxic to man, and a number of human deaths have been recorded where slurry agitation has occurred. At post-mortem examination, signs are non-specific, although pulmonary oedema is the most consistent finding.

Fire

Death of pigs in confined accommodation as a result of fire is all too common. Most deaths are associated with smoke asphyxiation and survivors will often subsequently grow very poorly. Obviously, some animals will also be burnt to death. Causes of farm fires include:

1. Non-specific electrical faults.
2. Arson.

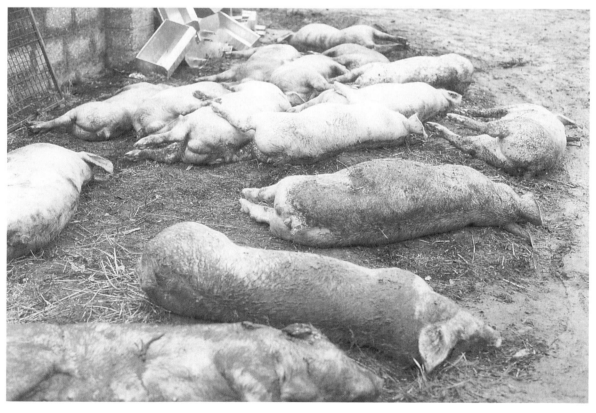

Fig. 132 Fire can kill pigs both by asphyxiation and burning.

3. Disturbance of creep lamps by sows.
4. Lightbulb drop onto creep areas.
5. Carelessness (for example, unattended bonfires).
6. Straw stack fires (caused, for example, by broken glass).

Electrocution

Electrocution of pigs occurs in a range of circumstances, as follows:

1. Where an individual pig has chewed through electrical cable that has carelessly been allowed to dangle within its reach.
2. Where an electrical fault creates a situation in which metal stanchions (used as dry sow crates, farrowing crates or pen divisions) become live.
3. Lightning strike.

In cases of lightning strike or where an individual pig has directly contacted a main cable, burn marks will be evident on the body. This is less likely where metalwork has become live. Some animals will survive electrocution but will suffer bone fractures, the vertebrae and shoulder blade (scapula) being particularly vulnerable. The carcasses of electrocuted pigs will contain multiple haemorrhages in the heart, muscle and, in particular, the conjunctiva.

Great care should be taken in cases of suspected electrical contact as the carcass itself may remain live. Many cases of electrocution are genuine accidents, but individual deaths are also often the result of careless stockmanship whereby pigs are allowed access to electrical wires.

Unfortunately, death is an all too common feature of commercial pig farming. Many pigs that are found dead will have suffered from a range of ailments that can be identified only by post-mortem examination. On top of these problems, a number of conditions can commence and kill the pig so rapidly that such cases are regarded as 'sudden deaths'. Accurate diagnosis based upon post-mortem examination is essential if appropriate preventative strategies are to be applied.

CHAPTER TWELVE

Urinary Conditions

The urinary system is the body's waste-disposal unit. Blood is filtered through the kidneys, where nitrogenous waste in the form of urea is removed in solution from it to produce urine. This will then be passed into a storage chamber – the bladder – before being voluntarily voided via the urethra. Production of urine is vital to the fluid and salt balance of the body, so any dysfunction of the kidneys will upset this vital mechanism and can lead to rapid death.

CYSTITIS/PYELONEPHRITIS

Infection of the urinary tract as a result of ascending bacterial challenge is the most common significant ailment of the urinary system. It occurs most often in the sow owing to the wide bore of the female urethra, the short distance between the bladder and the urethral orifice, and the fact that sows frequently lie in heavily contaminated areas, allowing colonization of the vagina. Mating is also significant factor leading to infection.

The urinary system can be regarded as self-cleaning. As urine is voided, the bladder and urethra are flushed clean. The most significant factor leading to infection ascending the urethra is therefore a failure to urinate frequently. This may arise as a consequence of water shortage or simply a behavioural fault; sows in dry sow stalls fed once a day spend most of their time lying down and may empty their bladders only once or twice a day. This gives ample time for ascended faecal-based

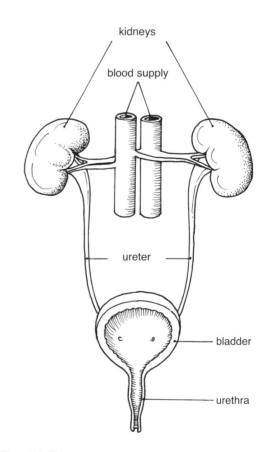

Fig. 133 Diagrammatic representation of the urinary system.

bacteria to colonize the bladder. The incidence of cystitis (and its more serious sequelae pyelonephritis) has reduced dramatically in the UK since the removal of confinement housing for dry sows, to the extent that it is

147

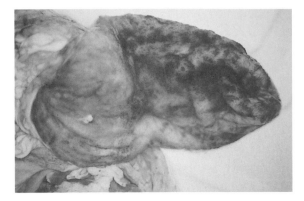

Fig. 134 *An inflamed and thickened bladder indicates cystitis.*

now an unusual clinical finding, although mild cystitis is still a common incidental finding at post-mortem examination.

Once cystitis has established, the sow may repeatedly strain and produce dribbles of urine. This may be cloudy or, in severe cases, even contain pus, mucus or blood. Body temperature is usually normal and appetite is unaffected. The bacteria involved in cystitis are most often common faecal contaminants such as *E. coli* and streptococci.

The effects of cystitis can be twofold. First, the pH of the urine may change, becoming more alkaline. This will favour the growth of some bacteria, in particular *Actinobaculum*

suis (formerly known as *Actinomyces suis, Corynebacterium suis* or *Eubacterium suis*), a commensal of the vagina of the sow and, particularly, the prepuce of the boar. Second, the flap valve system that exists to prevent backflow of urine up the ureter will be disturbed by thickening of the bladder wall, shortening the length of ureter within the wall. This shortening allows contaminated urine to ascend to the kidney, and if *A. suis* is present there infection will be acute and death will take place within hours. In the absence of *A. suis*, chronic pyelonephritis will occur, producing abscessation in the kidney. Passed urine will contain pus, blood and phosphate deposits, and there will be gradual weight loss and ultimately death or euthanasia. Slaughter of animals affected in this way often leads to carcass condemnation.

In acute pyelonephritis cases, the changes to the kidney may be minimal, although some pus may be seen in the pelvis of the kidney. This must be distinguished from purely phosphate deposits, which are commonly seen in normal sows. In chronic cases, abscessation and destruction of renal tissue, haemorrhage in the pelvic tissues, and blood and pus in the pelvis will be seen.

Outbreaks of cystitis and pyelonephritis can occur in herds, causing death in sows. Typically, acute pyelonephritis will be seen within

Fig. 135 *Illustration of bladder thickening due to cystitis and the effect on the uteral flap valve.*

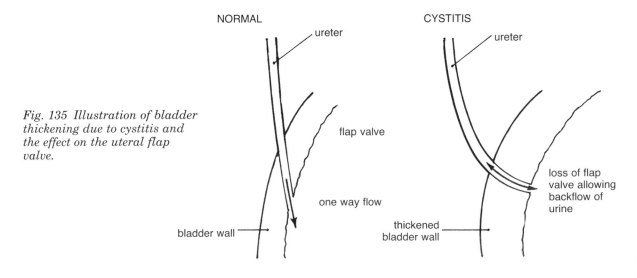

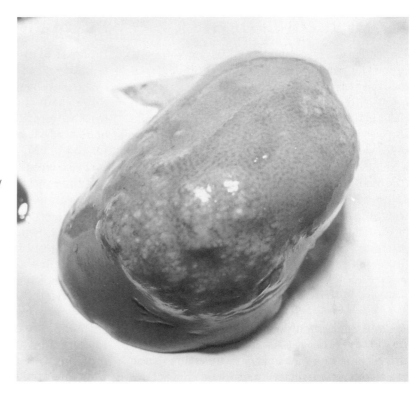

Fig. 136 Chronic abscessation/ necrosis that is typical of pyelonephritis.

a month of service, suggesting a venereal role for the disease.

Treatment and Control

Treatment of affected animals is often unsuccessful. In acute cases, the loss of renal function and the rise in blood potassium levels rapidly leads to heart failure. In chronic cases, once abscessation has occurred treatment is ineffective. Aggressive antibiotic treatment with broad-spectrum synthetic penicillin for five to seven days can be effective in early cases.

Prevention of disease is based upon hygiene, management and medication. Service pens and boar pens should be washed and disinfected regularly (this will help reduce ascending uterine infection, which many clinicians believe is linked to cystitis). The use of artificial insemination reduces the chance of venereal spread of *Actinobaculum suis*, and also avoids the risk of boars actually penetrating the urethra of the sow at mating. Increased urine flushing in the sow can be encouraged by adding salt to the feed (this will stimulate an increase in water intake), with attention to water availability at all stages. Where a herd problem occurs repeatedly, prevention can be effected through pulse medication of sows for three to four weeks every six months (or more frequently) with 1,000ppm oxytetracycline in feed.

UROLITHIASIS

The production of phosphate, urate or calcium carbonate deposits in urine is common (particularly in hard-water areas) but, unlike in most domestic species, the pig rarely experiences blockage of the ureter or urethra, even in the male. On rare occasions, these crystals will block the urethra of the young boar pig, leading to complete urinary obstruction and rapid death. The castrated male pet pig may be more at risk as a result of unusual diet and, if diagnosed early, can be treated by urethrotomy/urethrostomy in the same way as a dog.

GLOMERULONEPHRITIS

The filtration mechanism within the kidney is called the glomerulus. This allows small particles such as urea and dissolved salts to pass into the urine but prevents loss of larger particles such as blood proteins and cells. Damage can occur to the glomeruli as a result of allergic reactions to previous infections (for example, porcine dermatitis nephropathy syndrome; *see* Chapter 10), such that they leak protein. The urine will 'froth' on contact with the ground, weight loss will occur and the low blood protein levels that result will lead to oedema (fluid swelling) in the hind legs. Death will result from emaciation or acute renal failure.

CYSTS

Cysts are commonly found in pigs' kidneys at slaughter and may be of inherited origin (they can be part of a more extensive cystic process affecting the uterus, pancreas and other organs). Piglets can be born with cysts but further ones may form throughout life. They rarely cause clinical signs, although polycystic disease is fatal within a few days of life. Renal cysts normally constitute no more than incidental findings at post-mortem examination or meat inspection.

HYPERPLASTIC KIDNEYS

Absence of kidneys is an inherited congenital condition that is fatal. Pigs born with very small kidneys can survive a few weeks, growing poorly. Those completely lacking kidneys die within a few days of birth.

TUMOURS

Tumours are rare in pigs' kidneys and, when they do occur, are usually nephroblastomas, found incidentally at slaughter. Very rarely, renal carcinomas can occur and spread throughout the body, leading to progressive weight loss, signs dictated by affected tissues and, ultimately, death or euthanasia.

BLADDER OBSTRUCTION

Prolapse of the vagina, usually pre- or post-farrowing, can be complicated by involvement of the bladder. Straining causes the bladder to reflect into the prolapsed tissue, folding the urethra and blocking it so that urine cannot be voided. The ureters, however, continue to fill the bladder, which consequently becomes progressively enlarged.

If the condition goes untreated, back-flow of urine can lead to renal failure or, in extremes, the bladder will rupture following trauma. Death follows in both cases. If detected early enough, the bladder can be pushed back into position, but often it will be too full. In such instances, when it is not possible to catheterize the bladder, it must be drained by insertion of a 16-gauge needle under sterile conditions. Once it has been reduced in size sufficiently, it can be pushed back into place and the prolapse repaired.

The urinary system is concerned with maintaining the body's fluid balance and removing waste products. Abnormalities seen in the pig that affect the urinary system are relatively straightforward but, as with many other diseases in the commercial farming situation, the first recognized signs may well be death.

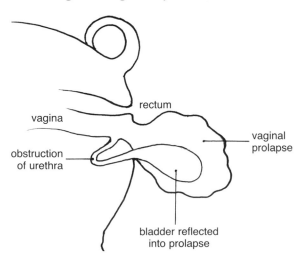

Fig. 137 Diagrammatic representation of vaginal prolapse with entrapped bladder.

CHAPTER THIRTEEN

Exotic Diseases

In 1924, following an outbreak of cattle plague (rinderpest) in Belgium that arose from the importation of zebus from India, twenty-eight countries signed an international agreement to monitor and control a range of specific economically damaging diseases of animals that had the potential to spread from country to country. The organization set up to carry out this task was the Office International des Épizooties (OIE, or World Animal Health Organisation). Today, the OIE consists of more than 160 member states, which contribute information on the incidence of nominated diseases. On the basis of this information, documentation produced by the OIE and made available to all members is used to restrict the movement of animals between countries and continents, and hence reduce the spread of disease.

Up until 2004, the OIE published two lists of diseases, A and B, categorizing animal diseases according to how fast they spread and the seriousness of their impact. List A consisted of diseases that have the potential for serious and rapid spread irrespective of national borders, have serious economic and/or public health complications, and are important in international trade in animals and animal products. Those that are relevant to pigs are listed below:

1. Foot and mouth disease.
2. Swine vesicular disease.
3. Classical swine fever.
4. African swine fever.
5. Vesicular stomatitis.

List A also contained diseases that, while not causing infection in the pig, have implications for trade in pigs:

1. Highly pathogenic avian influenza. There is potential for influenza viruses to cross species and recombine, and the pig is a potential 'factory' for highly pathogenic avian strains. Outbreaks of avian influenza lead to severe restrictions on pig movements.
2. Where non-pig diseases occur in a region or country, the controls on movement and trade imposed have implications for the pig. For example, in Europe, bluetongue in sheep leads to 100km (60-mile) exclusion zones where no animal movement is permitted.

As can be seen, the criteria for deciding whether a disease should be on List A included the propensity to spread by methods that are difficult or impossible to control. Examples of different methods of spread are given in Figure 138.

OIE List B included diseases of socio-economic and/or public health importance within countries that are significant for international trade – in other words, diseases that show a lower propensity to spread in uncontrollable ways. Diseases relevant to the pig are given below:

1. Anthrax.
2. Atrophic rhinitis.
3. Aujeszky's disease.
4. Leptospirosis.

Method of spread	Disease examples
Infected asymptomatic animals (normal trade)	All
Illegal trade	All
Infected meat	Classical swine fever
Human travel movements	African swine fever
Wind	Foot and mouth disease
Semen/ova	Classical swine fever
Bio-terrorism	All

Fig. 138 Spread of infectious diseases across national borders.

5. Porcine brucellosis.
6. Porcine cysticercosis.
7. Porcine reproductive and respiratory syndrome (PRRS).
8. Rabies.
9. Teschen disease.
10. Transmissible gastroenteritis (TGE).
11. Trichurisellosis.
12. Tuberculosis.

Based upon the principles of the OIE listings, individual states or collections of states (such as the European Union) draw up their own rules for the monitoring of specific disease and the action that should be taken if they are suspected. As an example, in the UK, the Department of Environment, Food and Rural Affairs (DEFRA) polices the Animal Health Act 1981, which lists a range of diseases relevant to the pig that are specifically notifiable and for which control programmes (such as slaughter policy) exist. These are listed below:

1. African swine fever.
2. Anthrax.
3. Aujeszky's disease.
4. Classical swine fever.
5. Foot and mouth disease.
6. Rabies.

7. Swine vesicular disease.
8. Teschen disease.
9. Vesicular stomatitis

The OIE also maintains something of a watching brief on a range of other animal diseases that appear from time to time around the world. These diseases have implications for both humans and animals, and include Japanese B encephalitis and Nipah virus. While such diseases are not specifically listed within the UK's Animal Health Act 1981 as being notifiable, the Act does give a minister of state the power to add any animal disease to the list should it be suspected in the country. Similar rules exist within the EU binding member states.

An additional source of information on infectious and exotic diseases in animals, though primarily relating to those that have an impact on human health (zoonoses) is the World Health Organisation (WHO). The website addresses for both WHO and the OIE are given in the Bibliography at the end of this book; readers should refer to these to monitor the changing disease picture around the world and the political decisions that will dictate the approach to them. Reference to the clinical effects of most of the diseases referred to above can be found elsewhere in the book (*see* Index).

CHAPTER FOURTEEN

Conditions Specific to Outdoor Pigs

Pigs kept out of doors, be it in backyards, large commercial production units or even in woodland, are susceptible to most of the ailments described in the earlier chapters. A range of the conditions already covered, such as sunburn, clostridial disease and phenol poisoning (through eating clay pigeons), are more likely to be seen outdoors than in housed animals, but there is also a small number of ailments that tend to be seen only in pigs kept out of doors (including pet pigs and wild boar).

LUNGWORM

Metastrongylus apri is a pig-specific parasite with an indirect life cycle that incorporates the earthworm. Therefore, the disease is seen only in pigs that have access to soil. The developing and adult worms live in the bronchi (airways) of the pig, particularly in diaphragmatic lobes of the lungs, having migrated there from the intestine. (Their migration through liver can lead to large white spots that are distinct from milk spots associated with *Ascaris suum* infection – *see* page 69.)

Coughing and loss of growth are the principal clinical signs, and at post-mortem examination pallor of the caudal diaphragmatic lobes of the lung is evident along with emphysema. Larvae and adult worms (up to 5cm/2in long) can be expressed from the cut surface of the lung, and eggs may be detected in the faeces of infected individuals using standard flotation techniques (unlike ruminant lungworm, which excrete larvae that require special techniques to detect). Occasionally, lungworm may be part of a complex respiratory disease picture with bacterial or viral involvement.

As with many parasitic worms, a balance is reached in adults where a low level of parasites maintains a reservoir of infections without clinical signs. Moreover, infected earthworms can persist for two to three years in the soil and so act as a long-term source of the parasite.

Treatment

Lungworm can be treated using either oral or injectable anthelmintics, but removal of the pigs from infected pasture is also needed to prevent reinfection. It should be remembered that, where pigs are infected with lungworm, it is highly likely that they will also have exposure to enteric worms and so multiple infections are common. At the time of writing, anthelmintic resistance is not a major issue in pig parasites.

STONE AND SAND COLIC

Sows kept out of doors tend to chew stones. The reasons for this are unclear, but it has been suggested that it is a vice resulting from inadequate gut fill. That said, the habit is seen in sows with ample access to grass and straw. Many of the stones are swallowed, and small ones pass through the intestine and can be seen in faeces. Larger ones tend to accumulate in the stomach, so that sows can be heard to rattle when they run. Many outdoor sows will show evidence of stones as incidental finding at slaughter or post-mortem examination. Occasionally, the stomach or intestine may rupture, particularly if flints have been ingested.

Additionally, outdoor sows will swallow large quantities of sand, picked up during feeding and rooting. Again, when ingested in modest quantities this is passed in faeces, but occasional sows will accumulate sand, particularly in the caecum, and this can ultimately lead to an impaction of the intestine. In commercial pig production, this condition may not be noticed and the sow will ultimately die (or be euthanized) following a period of weight loss. In the pet pig, failure to void faeces and abdominal distension may be noticed and the condition can be treated.

Treatment
Liquid paraffin drenches can remove sand impaction over a period of forty-eight hours (up to 4ltr [7pts] of liquid paraffin may be needed in total) but, if this is unsuccessful, surgical intervention is indicated.

FROSTBITE

Rarely seen, frostbite of the limbs occasionally occurs in young piglets in harsh weather conditions. The animal will initially be severely lame, with swelling and purple discoloration of a lower limb. If the condition is left to progress, the blood supply is completely occluded and a dry gangrene results, with ultimate loss of the affected tissue.

Treatment
Submersion of discoloured limbs in warm water (40–50°C/100–120°F) may reverse the early signs of frostbite, but if gangrene has occurred euthanasia is essential.

BALLOON FRIGHT

While it is not a disease, balloon fright is a well-recognized problem facing commercial outdoor pig producers. For reasons that are not clear, pigs react dramatically to hot-air balloons flying low over them. They will tend to stampede through wire fences and can be extremely difficult to recapture. Some sows so affected do not respect electrified wire in the future, which renders management of the herd extremely difficult. These animals will require culling. The effect of the fright and resulting stampede can also lead to abortion and dramatic effects on reproduction, with large numbers of sows returning to service (at both regular and irregular intervals).

Prevention
Outdoor pig units should not be set up close to established hot-air balloon launch sites, and liaison is needed with local balloon clubs to discourage pilots from flying low or close to outdoor pig units. As an interesting observation, pigs generally show little or no reaction to either fixed-wing or helicopter aircraft that fly low over them.

PLANT POISONING

Clearly, pigs kept outdoors have access to a wide range of vegetation not available to housed animals. Backyard- and woodland-based pigs in particular will come across a wide range of plants that are potentially poisonous, including pigweed (*Amaranthus* spp.), cocklebur (*Xanthium* spp.), clover (containing oestrogens), deadly nightshade and lupins. Readers should consult specific texts on plant poisons for more details. However, one specific condition in pigs resulting from plant poisoning warrants further description here.

In outdoor commercial pig farming, pigs form part of the rotation on an arable farm. On light land, it is not uncommon for pigs to follow crops of the Umbelliferae family, such as parsnips and carrots. These plants may contain photodynamic agents, which induce photosensitization of the white parts of the skin of the pig. Animals that have eaten them may appear stiff or lame owing to intense soreness of the skin (not unlike severe sunburn), but, over a period

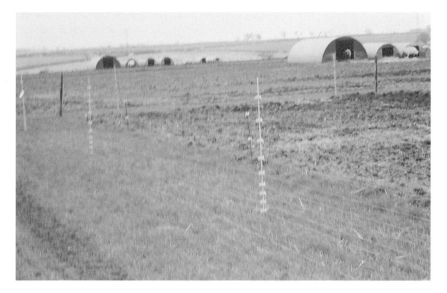

Fig. 139 Fox fencing can be essential for the outdoor pig farm.

of one to three days, a wet eczema develops that then dries and cracks to become intensely pruritic. Ultimately, the skin will become necrotic and slough off. In severe and untreated cases, death can occur, while in affected lactating sows, litter desertion is likely. Other crops that may cause photosensitivity include lucerne (alfalfa), rape, oats and clover.

Treatment

Removal of affected animals from both the vegetation and sunlight will allow healing, although in severe cases this can take several weeks.

PREDATION

Outdoor pigs – particularly young piglets – are vulnerable to predation by a number of wild animals. These can range from birds of prey (eagles and buzzards in particular) to foxes, dogs, wolves and even occasionally badgers. Foxes present the major hazard in most outdoor pig-production systems in the UK, but are often blamed for losses in farrowing paddocks without evidence. High electrified fencing incorporating seven to ten strands of wire is needed to keep foxes and other predators out of farrowing areas, as shown in Figure 139.

The commercial farming of pigs outdoors is a specialist division of the global pig industry and is suited only to specific locations. However, many pet, backyard and smallholding pig-keeping enterprises expose the animal to outdoor conditions from which most indoor farmed pigs are isolated. It is, therefore, necessary to be aware of the few conditions that are largely unique to the outdoor situation by virtue of the pigs' exposure to vegetation, soil, the weather and wildlife.

Bibliography

For readers who wish to extend their knowledge beyond the scope of this book generally, or who require greater detail regarding any specific conditions, the following books, periodicals and websites are recommended.

BOOKS

Straw, B.E., D'allaire, S., Mengeling, W.L., and Taylor, D.J. (eds), *Diseases of Swine*, 8th edn (Blackwell Science, 1999).

Ministry of Agriculture, Fisheries and Food, *British Poisonous Plants*, MAFF Bulletin 161 (HMSO, 1968).

Muirhead, M.R., and Alexander, T.J.L., *Managing Pig Health and the Treatment of Disease* (S.M. Enterprises, 1997).

Smith, W.J., Taylor, D.J., and Penny, R.H.C., *Colour Atlas of Diseases and Disorders of the Pig* (Wolfe Publishing Ltd, 1999).

Straw, B.E., D'allaire, S., Mengeling, W.L., and Taylor, D.J. (eds), *Diseases of Swine*, 8th edn (Blackwell Science Ltd, 1999).

Taylor, D.J. (ed.), *Pig Diseases*, 7th edn (Blackwell Publishing, 1999).

JOURNALS

In Practice (Journal of Veterinary Postgraduate Clinical Studies).
Journal of Swine Health and Production.
Pig Journal.

Websites

Department of Environment, Food and Rural Affairs (UK):
www.defra.gov.uk/animalh/animihdx.htm
Office International des Épizooties (World Animal Health Organisation): www.oie.int
Pig Diseases Information Centre:
www.pighealth.com
The Pig Site: www.ThePigSite.com
Pig Veterinary Society (UK):
www.pigvetsoc.org.uk
World Health Organisation: www.who.int/en

Glossary

Acclimatization The process of exposing incoming animals to the microbial population of a farm in a controlled way.

Acute A sudden-onset or rapid-acting condition.

Anoestrus A failure in the oestrus cycle.

Anoxia Total lack of oxygen.

Artesia ani The absence of an anus.

Ataxia Loss of control, usually of the back legs, when a 'wobbling' gait is created.

Atrophy Wasting of tissue.

Brown fat An energy-dense tissue (lacking in the pig).

Catabolism The abnormal breakdown of tissues that occurs where there is a shortage of energy to supply bodily needs.

Caudal Rear or hind end.

Chemosis Swollen eyelids.

Chronic A long-standing or slowly developing condition.

Congenital Present at birth.

Cranial Front or head end.

Dorsal The back.

Dysentery Diarrhoea containing fresh blood.

Dyspnoea Disturbed or laboured breathing.

Dystocia Interruption to parturition.

ELISA (enzyme-linked immunosorbent assay) A laboratory test used to detect antibodies or antigens (microbes) in a sample.

Emphysema The abnormal presence of air pockets within tissues. When it occurs in the lungs, it equates to overinflation.

Encephalitis Inflammation of the brain.

Endometritis Inflammation of the endometrium, or inner lining of the uterus.

Epistaxis Haemorrhage from the nasal chambers.

Euthanasia Humane destruction.

Feedback The technique of exposing animals – particularly breeding gilts – to infected material such as faeces from other animals to promote immunity. It is a crude form of vaccination.

Flushing The technique of increasing energy intake in sows prior to service.

Haemorrhage Leakage of blood from vessels.

Histopathology The microscopic changes that occur in tissues during disease processes.

Hypoxia Partial lack of oxygen.

Ileo-caeco-colic valve The junction between the small and large intestines.

-itis When added as a suffix, indicates inflammation of part of the body – for example, arthritis is inflammation of the joint.

Lymphadenopathy The abnormal increase in size of lymph nodes (glands).

Mammogenesis Development of mammary tissue (udder) prior to farrowing.

Melaena Digested blood within faeces.

Meninges The protective sacs containing the brain.

Mummification The sterile partial reabsorption of a dead foetus *in utero*.

Neonate Newly born.

Neuro-endocrine system The control mechanism for physiological processes in the body, involving links between the nervous system and hormone production.

Nystagmus An uncontrolled flicking of the eyes within their sockets, characteristic of brain dysfunction.

Oestrus Standing heat.

Oestrus cycle The female reproductive cycle.

Opisthotonus Excessive extension of the head over the shoulders, which results in an affected pig falling over backwards.

Orchitis Inflammation of the testicles.

Ovulation The release of eggs from the ovary.

Parturition The process of giving birth (farrowing).

Pathogenesis The development of abnormality in the body (pathology) in response to disease challenge.

PCR (polymerase chain reaction) A precise laboratory test that detects part of the genetic material (DNA) of an organism (virus, bacteria and so on) and so is used to confirm its presence in a sample.

Peracute The very sudden onset of a condition.

Perinatal Occurring around and soon after birth.

Perineum The area under the tail including the anus, vulva, testicles and upper caudal surface of the hind legs.

Pheromone A chemical produced in the body of one animal that affects another.

Pleurisy Inflammation of the lining of the chest cavity (pleura), creating adhesion between the chest wall and the lungs.

Pyrexia Raised body temperature.

Scour Diarrhoea.

Steaming up The increase in nutrient intake prior to farrowing.

Systemic Affecting the whole body.

Trochanter The bony protruberances at the top of the thigh bone (femur), to which muscles attach.

Vas deferens The tubes connecting the testicles to the urethra.

Ventral Underside (belly).

Zoonotic A disease that can be transmitted to people from animals.

Index